PROCESSED FOOD ADDICT

Is This Me?

PROCESSED FOOD ADDICT

Is This Me?

Why You Can't Stop Eating
Junk Food and How to
Permanently Break
the Cycle of Yo-Yo Dieting,
Bingeing, and Starving

KARREN-LEE RAYMOND, PHD

Copyright © 2018 Raymond Family Trust—First edition 2019 All rights reserved.

Published by *KLWR Publications*
Brisbane, Queensland, Australia.

No part of this publication may be reproduced or transmitted in any form or by any means, electronic or mechanical, including photocopying, recording, or by an information storage and retrieval system, without prior written permission of the copyright owners.

This book is sold subject to the condition that it shall not, by way of trade or otherwise, be lent, resold, hired out, or otherwise circulated without the publisher's prior consent (*KLWR Publications, Australia*) in any form of binding or cover other than that in which it is published, including this condition being imposed on the subsequent purchaser. Under no circumstances may any part of this book be photocopied for resale.

This is a work of non-fiction. Case studies, names, and identifying details (unless written consent has been given) have been changed to protect the privacy of individuals. The case studies shared are typical and born out of experience of working many years with people requiring processed food addiction treatment and recovery.

ISBN: 978-0-6468362-0-1 (Hardcover)
ISBN: 978-0-6484362-4-9 (Paperback)
ISBN: 978-0-6484362-5-6 (e-book)

Editing by Nina Shoroplova | NinaShoroplova.ca
Book Formatting by AmitDey | amitdey2528@gmail.com

HEALTH DISCLAIMER

The information provided in this book is not a substitute for medical advice, diagnosis, or treatment, nor is it to be construed as such. While all attempts are made to present accurate information, the information may not be appropriate for your specific circumstances and may become outdated over time. The basic eating regime proposed to eliminate processed foods provides information for beginning to phase out and fundamentally eliminate processed foods. This basic eating regime is intended for those individuals eighteen years and over. I cannot guarantee that the information provided in this book will continue to reflect the most up-to-date medical research. Information is provided without any representations or warranties of any kind. Please consult a qualified addiction specialist for medical advice, and always seek the advice of a qualified healthcare provider with any questions you may have regarding your health, diet, and nutritional program. Furthermore, this book does not assume any liability with regard to health results based on the use of the information provided here. Lastly, advertisers, commenters, and linked sites are solely responsible for their views and content and do not necessarily represent the views of Processed Food Addict: Is This Me? Typically, before starting any new health regimes, please consult with a medical health professional.

To

*Geoff P. Lovell, PhD,
in gratitude*

Contents

Another Doctor's Opinion. xv
Preface xix
Acknowledgments xxiii
To the Reader xxv

Chapter One: My Professional Perspective on Processed
                 Food Addiction. 1
Processed Food Addiction. 6
    Can You Identify? 6
        Pamela Shares. 6
        Donna Shares 6
        Jane Shares 6
        Miranda Shares 9
        Joyce Shares. 11
    Processed Food Addict, Alcoholic, Drug Addict,
    Nicotine Addict, Codependent, Substance Abuser?. 12
        Let's Share. 13
        The Term "Processed Food Addiction". 14
        Let's Share. 17

Chapter Two: Questions, Questions, Questions 21
    Let's Share. 23
    Olivia Shares 24
    Angela Shares 24
    Let's Share. 25
  On the Other Hand … 26
    Janice Shares 27
  I Thought I Was … 30
    Jenny Shares 32
    Dianna Shares 32
  I Know I'm Different 34
    Josephine Shares. 40
    Let's Share. 46
    Let's Share. 48

Chapter Three: A Paradigm of the Phases of Processed Food
                    Addiction 51
  Processed Food Addiction: An Analogy 51
  Where Are You in This Stormy Sea? 53
    Exposure and/or Vulnerability to Addiction 54
    Maureen Shares 54
    Jill Shares 54
    The Inquisitive Eater 55
    Joan Shares 55
    The Social and/or Emotional Eater 56
    The Controlling Eater-cum-Health Fanatic 57
    The Recreational Eater 60
    Bella's Case Study. 61

Impulsive Eater. 62
   Katrina's Case Study. *63*
   Rosie *64*
   Angie *65*
Psychological Dependence. 66
   A Case Study *69*
   Jess. *70*
   Emily *71*
Compulsive Eater *73*
   Case Study *74*
Crossing the Invisible Line into Addiction *76*

Chapter Four: A Non-PFA Versus a PFA *81*
   The Case of Joy, a Non-PFA. *81*
   The Case of Caryn, a Severe Processed Food Addict 82

Chapter Five: Grief and Recovery 89
The Five Stages of Grief 89
   Denial 89
   Anger 92
      Francine Shares About Anger 94
   Bargaining 94
      Penny Shares About Bargaining 96
   Depression 96
      Amanda's Case Study *97*
   Last but Definitely Not Least ... Acceptance. 98

Chapter Six: Abstinence with Peace of Mind 99
   Case Study *102*

Chapter Seven: Consequences of Processed Food Addiction . . . 105
    Withdrawal 105
        Beth Shares *106*
    Tolerance 109
        Betty Shares *110*
        Fiona Shares *110*
        Leah Shares *111*
        Annie Shares *111*
        Heidi Shares *112*
    The Empty Processed Food Addict Syndrome 113
        Kylie Shares *115*
    Submission Versus Surrender 116
    Multi-comorbidity 117

Chapter Eight: Changing Addiction Diagnoses and Treatments . . 119
    A Family Disease 120
    Intervention 123
        1. Spiritual Insight 124
        2. Nutritional Hygiene 126
        3. Self-Help Group 127
    A Threefold Disease 128
    Physical 128
        Olivia Shares *130*
        Mia Shares *130*
    Mental 131
        Joanna Shares *133*
        Amelia Shares *135*

A Devilish Alter Ego: The Ignoble Personality of Addiction. . . . 138
   Jennifer Shares. *140*
   Nelly Shares *142*
   Naomi Shares *143*
Powerlessness. 146
   A Spiritual Solution 147
   Nora Shares. *148*

Chapter Nine: Touching on Relapse. 155
   Let's Wind Up This Portion for Now 159

Chapter Ten: Recovery Begins 161
Preliminary Elimination of Processed Foods 169
   Grace Shares *170*
   Jane Shares *171*
   Christine Shares. *171*
Preliminary Baseline for the Elimination
of Processed Foods 174
   A Basic List of Non-Processed Food Products 175
      Protein *175*
      Fruit. *175*
      Salad *175*
      Cooked Vegetables *175*
      Carbohydrates. *176*
      Dairy *176*
      Oils, Salad Dressings, and Accompaniments *176*
      Sauces *176*
      Herbs, Seasonings, Spices *176*

>> ***Condiments*** 177
>> ***Broth*** 177
>> Guidelines for Men 177

Chapter Eleven: Stories of Recovery 179
> Stories to Share 181
>> ***Julia's Expedition*** 181
>> ***Liz's Voyage*** 186
>> ***Lee's Odyssey*** 192
>> ***Jacinta's Journey*** 198
>> ***Rob Remembers*** 204
>> ***Sheri's Crusade*** 208
>> ***Janice's Jaunt*** 217
>> ***Shandell Shares*** 225
>> ***Betty's Bio*** 230
>> ***Karen's Case*** 237

Afterword 243

Appendix A: 12-Step Self-Help Groups 247

Appendix B: CDs, DVDs, Literature, Services, and Products in the Broad Field of Addiction 248

Appendix C: Country Help Lines 249
> Australia 249
> Canada 249
> UK 249
> USA 250

Glossary **251**
Bibliography **261**
About the Author **265**
    Contact 267
    Recent Publications 267

Another Doctor's Opinion[1]

Donald J. Kurth, MD

In 1935, a New York stockbroker and an Akron, Ohio, physician came together to unlock the perplexing malady of addiction and alcoholism for the many millions who suffered across the globe. Over many years, the secrets to treating this and many other addictive diseases have found successful application in the treatment of both substance and behavioral addictions. A bit of background might put all this into perspective.

Bill Wilson, the New York stockbroker, had begun his drinking career as many do, integrating alcohol into his personal and professional life as a pleasant diversion and a social lubricant. For some time, it seemed that there were no negative consequences to Bill's drinking activities. He attracted lots of friends, found a lovely wife and married, and succeeded in business. Bill had arrived! He was poised on the verge of even more business and financial success. He crushed the difficulties life threw at him, moving forward to even greater successes in the face of adversity.

In just a few short years, though, his alcohol-related scrapes increased and his life successes faded away. Financial troubles

---

[1] This foreword is so named because in *Alcoholics Anonymous*, William Duncan Silkworth, MD, wrote a passage he named "The Doctor's Opinion."

ensued. Soon Bill's health began to fail and the wolf was at the doorstep. Steady job prospects evaporated and he began stealing money from his wife's purse just to obtain the alcohol he needed on a daily basis. Bill developed a pattern of hospitalizations and relapses, and he soon began to fear that permanent commitment to a hospital for alcoholics might be the only option for his survival.

During one episode at Towns Hospital in New York, Bill met the renowned physician William Silkworth. Dr. Silkworth explained to Bill that his addiction to alcohol was not a moral failing or a character defect but rather a disease—an allergy of the body, coupled with an obsession of the mind. Shortly after discharge, Bill relapsed again. About this time, he was contacted by Ebby Thacker, an alcoholic high school chum. To Bill's surprise, his old friend showed up sober. Ebby explained to Bill that he had found a spiritual solution and that by applying certain principles he had been able to achieve sustained sobriety. Although Bill continued to drink for some time following his reunion with Ebby, he was deeply impressed with his old friend's success. Bill began to think that perhaps he, too, could achieve sobriety through application of these principles.

Upon returning for his third visit to Towns Hospital, Bill presented his ideas to Dr. Silkworth, who supported them wholeheartedly. He explained to Bill that a psychic change, coupled with working with others who suffered as he did, might be the only course that could help Bill. Thus, Bill began his quest for a solution. He soon met Bob Smith, MD, in Akron, Ohio, and together, "Bill W and Dr. Bob" began to approach others who suffered from alcoholism, asking them to share their personal experiences, strength, and hope. Soon, a small but dedicated group formed in Ohio and another soon after that in New York. After some early struggles, during which the twelve steps were identified, Alcoholics Anonymous began to grow and flourish, numbering now over two million members worldwide.

Remember, these pioneers were hopeless alcoholics with no clinical training and no road map, carrying a message of recovery to others who suffered as they once had.

As word of the success of Alcoholics Anonymous spread, others recognized the power that Bill and Bob had unleashed and began to apply these principles to a broad range of addictive diseases. And it worked. Across the globe there are now dozens of twelve-step groups, each with its own addiction focus, but all applying the same set of spiritual principles to achieve their own brand of sobriety.

The personal experience and clinical focus of Karren-Lee Raymond, PhD, have been in the area of processed food addiction. In her chosen field, Dr. Raymond is arguably one of the most knowledgeable in the world. She has been my friend and colleague for many years, and I have been honored to have a front row seat as she developed her ideas and attracted a following of those who have suffered as she once did before finding her way to recovery.

I certainly cannot tell you that you are (or are not) a processed food addict. But if you think you might be, or if you identify with the examples provided in *Processed Food Addict: Is This Me?*, then take a few moments to read through the explanations and examples Dr. Raymond presents in such masterly detail. See if some of these experiences apply to you as well; then, perhaps, you may discover you are not alone, and this book may even help you to find peace of mind and a better way of life. I wish you all the best in your endeavor.

Donald J. Kurth, MD, MBA, MPA
Medical Director, Social Model Recovery Systems, Los Angeles, California
Chief of Addiction Medicine (Retired), Behavioral Medicine Center, Loma Linda University
Associate Professor (Retired), Loma Linda University, Loma Linda, California
Fellow of the International Society of Addiction Medicine
Distinguished Fellow of the American Society of Addiction Medicine (DFASAM)
Past President, ASAM
Former Mayor, City of Rancho Cucamonga, California

Preface

For centuries, people have been putting ink to paper, which is the keystone of passing on ideas and knowledge from past generations to future generations. Hence, people have many reasons for writing books. Mine are simply based on a belief, and on my personal and clinical experience, that processed food addiction (PFA) is a chronic illness, analogous to alcoholism and other substance use disorders (SUDs).

Thus, I was encouraged to write this book to help open the eyes and ears of people of all races, creeds, colors, and vocations. Too often, a person feels stigmatized by having an addiction. Hence, I am inviting you to help create a bridge of unity and understanding, continuing to use alcohol- and drug-addiction models as a baseline, so we can find common footing.

So, I have written a book of insight, of knowledge, of hope, and of wisdom. I want to share this book with as many people as possible, explaining my beliefs about, and my experiences with, this disease that is founded in denial, unbeknown to the processed food addict. It is based predominantly on what I have learned and continue to learn in the clinic, through research, from others, from my own experiences, and through what I have learned globally from a large number of professionals I respect as experts in the field of "addiction medicine," as it is becoming more widely known today.

However, the central reason I write is to share with you that I have personal experience with the disease of processed food addiction (PFA). I too have lived a life of always being told what my problem was but never finding a solution. I went from anorexia and bulimia clinics to international jaunts, desperately trying to find an answer to my problems. Not to mention the times I was in various psychiatric wards due to misdiagnoses, including depressive disorder, bipolar disorder, schizophrenia, and obsessive-compulsive disorder (just to name a few). This ultimately led to my attempted suicide at age twenty-one. I would have done anything to stop the mental and physical torture of an unknown and untreated (and seemingly untreatable) disease.

This is now a disease I have researched extensively, both professionally and personally—the phenomenon of processed food addiction.

My recovery began when I learned, understood, and accepted that alcoholism was a disease. A light went on within me, and I knew I had the undiscovered solution to a disease that needed to be unveiled to the world. Before that, little did I know that I too had the same craving phenomenon for processed foods that an alcoholic has for alcohol. Thus began one long journey to find and establish *my* recovery from a progressive and fatal disease.

Many individuals from the professional medical arena and the clergy and many recovered alcoholics, drug addicts, and non-professionals have been instrumental in helping me. They understood the medical model of addiction and knew I was not a bad person trying to *get good*, but a very sick person (a young woman who should have been in the prime of her life) trying to survive in a world that had little knowledge or understanding of her disease. Through my extensive personal, and later academic and professional, education and research, I came to understand nothing was *wrong* with me; I just had an untreated, unknown public health and social problem—processed food addiction.

In my twenties, I was placed in a rehabilitation center for addiction. This was the inception of the unique understanding that skyrocketed me to pursue and understand the disease of processed food addiction in its varied facets—just like any other addiction. I had tried every known behavioral, psychological, and self-help program, and diets ad infinitum, to beat this thing, but to no avail.

Miraculously, I was spiritually guided to the individuals who were continually placed in my path. They encouraged me to pursue this gift and passion of insight to an unknown global malady. A malady that I have personally and professionally brought to the forefront in the medical, academic, clinical, and social world.

Hence, as the pioneer in the diagnosis and treatment of and recovery from processed food addiction, I say, may this book answer your many questions, give you and your families much sought-after hope, love, and understanding that you too are not alone; you too can recover from a seemingly hopeless state of body, mind, and spirit. Finally, I dedicate this book to you.

May you be so bold and brave as to ask yourself, "Is this me?"

The global message I present here is simply this: the disease of processed food addiction is a reality. It can be successfully treated, and most processed food addicts can recover and go on to lead a life of happiness, productivity, and usefulness. Most importantly, their lives can be free of the craving underpinned by the mental twist and championed by a seductiveness that remains hidden until ... until one reaches out for help.

The disease of addiction is the only disease I know that tells the patient they do not have a disease. (I use the label *patient*, as I am a practitioner, treating individuals suffering from the disease of addiction.) Hence, the disease concept provides processed food addicts with much-needed answers, bringing about the most extraordinary news (once again) that the processed food addict is not a bad person trying to be good—but a sick person trying to get well. Their thinking and actions may be immoral while under the influence of processed food, but the disease is not their fault.

I truly believe what was shared with me early on in my training in the field of addiction: The heart and soul of recovery from addiction is accepting the disease concept of addiction. This is a message of understanding, of acceptance, and of hope.

> *May the light of knowledge surround us,*
>
> *May the love of God enfold us,*
>
> *May the integrity of passion enlighten us,*
>
> *May the humility of doing God's work embolden us,*
>
> *May we keep steadfast on the path,*
>
> *May we free the world of addictive substances,*
>
> *May we love others unconditionally,*
>
> *May we have the courage to do the next right thing always*
>
> *No matter how difficult,*
>
> *AND ... may we help uncover the wonderful human beings that God created*
>
> *By clearing their minds and bodies of addictive substances.*

Lastly, I would like to share with you a little saying I made up in the early days of treating the disease of processed food addiction. It is something I use on a daily basis in treatment: "Abstinence with peace of mind is the norm for a processed food addict."

Warmly,
Karren-Lee Raymond

Acknowledgments

I would like to thank all the patients, and their families, whom I have worked with over several decades in the addiction realms—initially in the alcoholism and drug addiction field of addiction medicine. My early work led me to apply similar procedures and methodologies in the processed food addiction world. I have been thrilled to watch your eyes shine and to be the benefactor of your feeling overjoyed, thrilled to finally hear *your* voices full of confidence, and thrilled to realize you have regained an inner knowing of your own usefulness and purpose. You continue to journey through the stages of life as the disease of addiction moves into remission and the "subtle voice dissipates."

William Shakespeare wrote: "All the world's a stage, and all the men and women merely players: they have their exits and their entrances; and one man in his time plays many parts, his acts being seven ages."

We are each marching to the beat of our own drum, one day at a time.

I would not know where to begin if I were to acknowledge the guidance and wisdom of so, so many people from the medical and mental health fields, religious circles in all their different movements, and those everyday individuals in the many and varied roles they play in society. From those who have crossed my path for a short period of time, who provided me with the knowledge and motivation to keep pursuing this path, to the persons I frequently came into contact with.

If I have seen further than others, it is by standing upon the shoulders of giants. I hope the many people who have helped me to create this book but are too many to name will understand that the limiting factor is the lack of space, and not a lack of gratitude.

To the Reader

Any quotations and case histories in this book are based on the actual experiences and thoughts of real people, used with permission. However, some names and distinguishing details have been changed in order to protect the confidentiality of these persons. In chapter 11, however, these individuals have chosen to keep their first names while sharing their case histories.

When discussing processed food addicts in general terms, for this writing I have perhaps used the pronouns *she* and *her* more often. This is only for simplicity, and ease of reading.

PROCESSED FOOD ADDICT

IS THIS ME?

CHAPTER ONE

My Professional Perspective on Processed Food Addiction

Processed food addiction and its secondary complications—including obesity, type 2 diabetes (t2d), mental health issues, disordered eating practices, cardiac disease, hypertension, cancer, dementia, and so on—represent one of, if not the most global, rampant, communicable diseases of the twenty-first century. Unfortunately, the "obesity epidemic" devilishly continues to grow as a major health risk at an alarming rate. Media daily highlights its global and continual rise in prevalence.

I was reading some statistics recently that highlight this rise: approximately 1.9 billion adults are overweight and an additional 650 million are obese (WHO, 2016). Despite the continual search for solutions to combat these trends, establishing public health models is challenging, to say the least, as we try to abate the obesity pandemic. I have watched and researched traditional and contemporary prevention approaches that have been implemented for decades, investigating the causes and consequences of obesity, including public health models, educational initiatives, counseling, diet and exercise plans, and of late, weight-loss surgery options. Over and over again (and I am confident I do not stand alone), I hear the continuing struggles of some individuals whose overweight is resistant to treatments, possibly because interventions do not address underlying causes such as processed food addiction—a cause that has really come to light only recently.

Most emphatically, I understand that an individual's role of free choice and self-will is not negated by the notion of addiction. However, as I treat processed food addicts and witness their return to health, it is becoming clearer and clearer that there is such a phenomenon as processed food addiction, which, for some people, underlies a powerlessness that the individual and society do not yet understand from an addiction perspective.

What I have seen in the clinic with the majority of patients is that as we treat the malady of addiction (by eliminating the cause—processed foods), the consequences (e.g., weight, depression, anxiety, type 2 diabetes, hypertension, and more) dissipate substantially over time. If only the consequences are treated, then the cause (processed food addiction) is still operational and will present again, sooner or later.

An addict may be classed as many things: weak-willed, gluttonous, stubborn, belligerent, and arrogant on the one hand, and on the other, sweet, nice, and innocent, as if butter wouldn't melt in her mouth. But she will ingest processed food not because she can, but because she is compelled to, which appears to be a supreme global paradox. Usually, when the processed food addict is "on a diet," just as an alcoholic goes "on the wagon," she feels in control—*until* the **uncontrollable craving (allergy)** to binge (or drink or use or ingest) rears up again. A physical allergy is a predisposition to restlessness, irritability, and discontentment (conscious or subconscious) that precedes a desire to ingest processed foods, a desire that is beyond the person's physical and mental control. The processed food addict's willpower is nonexistent when it comes to stopping themselves from ingesting processed foods, that is, bingeing (or drinking or using) again. Paradoxically, when hungover (from whatever substance), the addict will pray, beg, and hope in earnest to once again abstain (that is, eliminate the substance—processed foods), be sober (eliminate the alcohol), or go clean (eliminate the drugs).

Processed food addiction as I know and understand it is not a behavioral addiction, although like other substance addictions, it has behavioral components. As with other addictive substances, including alcohol and drugs, processed foods are chemically based. Yes, processed foods have been chemically enhanced, for example with monosodium glutamate, perhaps better known as MSG; artificial sweeteners; and high-fructose corn syrup, which is now a staple in a large variety of processed food items. Thus, the processed food addict is not addicted to the feeling experienced after ingesting but to the substance—the chemicals in the processed foods.

Ingesting processed food keeps an individual's blood sugar unstable, causing neurological confusion. It feeds symptoms such as depression, which in turn increases the person's desire for more processed food, making their life torture. This blood-sugar roller coaster that imprisons processed food addicts and holds them captive is remarkably similar to an alcoholic's symptoms during the withdrawal and sometimes post-withdrawal stages. (Interestingly enough, liquid alcohol, the intoxicating constituent of spirits, beer, and wine, is produced by the natural fermentation of sugars.) As the processed food addict ingests the processed food, her blood sugars immediately rise. This temporarily alleviates psychological symptoms, including depression, anxiety, stress, and mood swings. Hence, it is paramount that a potential processed food addict understand the disease of addiction—its biochemical nature. Then and only then can the addict be educated in how to protect themselves from the disease.

I am seeing more and more recovering alcohol and drug addicts in danger of relapse. Not because they are vulnerable or in denial regarding their addiction but because they are ingesting processed foods, which keeps the desire and craving for alcohol (and other substances) active. On the other hand, it is important to note not all addicts are addicted to processed food. However, I am seeing more and more addicts who successfully eliminated other substances months and years earlier finding their sobriety very challenging. They are the ones in danger of relapsing.

Society understands this phenomenon of processed food addiction the least of all the addictions. It is an utter inability to *not* ingest the substance—in this case, processed foods—no matter how much one might wish or try by one's own willpower. This demonstrates that processed food addiction is not about overcoming one's lack of control; it is about being powerless over an allergy that condemns one to ingest processed food even against one's will.

In fact, processed food addiction is not uniquely an issue of psychological control. Numerous patients have been on a diet or a weight-loss plan for several months, to enable them to solve a dilemma or to work toward a desired business opportunity that would have led to bigger and better opportunities later on. Then, prior to signing a contract that would have set them up financially, they ingested some processed food. The phenomenon of craving kicked in, hijacking the brain and overriding any ability to go through with the business arrangement. These people did not ingest the processed food in order to avoid facing the potential business opportunity; they were ingesting to overcome a craving outside their mental control.

The most pertinent question I get asked is "What are processed foods?" I suggest primarily that you ask yourself this question. Most of the processed food addicts I treat and work with could easily have aced any dietetics and nutrition course, especially with the amount of knowledge accumulated over the years (and in some cases, decades) of trying to work out how to *control* and *fix* their problems with food.

Broadly (and I emphasize *broadly*), over the past several decades *processed food* has typically come to refer to commercial products that have little or no nutritional value, have minimal vitamins and minerals, are very high in calories (kilojoules), and are loaded with fat, sugars, salt, and refined carbohydrates. The term *processed food* can be interchanged with *refined food* or *fast food*, meaning "ready-to-eat take-out food."

Literature abounds on the topic of discerning *junk food*, a label conceived in the mid-twentieth century. Some literature postulates that *junk food* was superseded by other labels, one being *cheat food*, used by an American doctor in a health column. Yes, there is an argument that most foods nowadays, whether natural, organic, or whatever, have been tampered with in some way, shape, or form. For further information, I encourage you to turn to chapter 7, which goes into this topic a little bit more in-depth.

Processed food addiction is a frightening, persistent disease, seductive in its approaches, deceitful in its onset, and all-encompassing in how it affects one's body, mind, and spirit. Its chameleon-like nature makes it challenging for people (general public and professionals alike) to put a finger on it. In its wake, it harms all who live with it and who come into contact with it, including family, friends, and work colleagues. Moreover, its causes continue to be controversial: Genetic? Environmental? Neurological? Mental illness? Sin? Vice? Disease? And the list goes on. Unfortunately, without a resolution, knowledge takes a back seat. For example, the disease's different labels—including *ultra-processed foods addiction, highly processed foods addiction, refined foods addiction, food addiction, compulsive overeating, chocaholism*—create a universal limitation.

At the end of the day, it is not the label that is dealt with but the disease itself, and as with alcoholism, the debate continues as to whether processed food addiction is a symptom, a social problem, or a disease of addiction. Do we treat it with a medical model or a social model? Indeed, alcoholism and addiction to drugs, nicotine, and other substances have all traveled down similar well-trodden paths.

Since the 1990s, I have had the privilege of serving professionally in the field of addiction, primarily in alcoholism and drug addiction, and in the last twenty years, I have focused more on the realm of processed food addiction. Over many years, it has been both my honor and my privilege to observe the disease in all its facets and under its many different labels.

Processed Food Addiction

Can You Identify?

Below, I share with you some typical stories I hear every day at work in my clinic. Can you identify with any of them? In addiction treatment and recovery we say, "Look for the similarities and not the differences."

Pamela Shares

> *If I could just lose these 13 lb. (7 kg.), then I will be beautiful enough, good enough, happy enough, and successful enough, and then I can eat what I want and be normal. The weight comes off, and then normal eating recommences only to find that the weight has been put back on, plus a few more pounds as a bonus—another attempt—another failure?? UGH!*

Donna Shares

> *This time it is going to be different, so I try a different diet, a different weight-loss program, food plan, personal trainer, plus I see a mental health clinician. I lose all the weight AGAIN, then resume eating normally and all the weight comes back on again plus a few extra pounds to add to the insanity.*

Jane Shares

> *Argh! All that hard work gone down the drain. BUT this time will be the last time I will ever have to diet. I have a special event coming up, so I must look fantastic for that. SECOND THOUGHT, I'LL WAIT UNTIL MONDAY! Then I get to have one last binge over the weekend and when Monday morning comes, I will start again. Lots of variables come into play in my mind—is Monday morning a specific date such as New Year's Day, Easter Monday (I should be sick of chocolate by then), Thanksgiving, my birthday,*

when I get pregnant, after the baby is born; when I get married; when I graduate? I'll wait until after that and then I will start.

I now have the diet and a new set of soldiers on board to help me reach my goal, including a new dietitian soldier and a nutritionist soldier. I've left the gym and now have a personal trainer soldier who also says she will motivate me; a new health-care professional to implement the latest psychological approach, such as mindfulness, Cognitive Behavior Therapy, to control my weight-loss problem. They are all lined up. How can I fail now? I am looking fabulous as the weight drops off—people are telling me how beautiful I am. This strengthens my resolve to keep going—then the big day arrives. "Goal weight." Yahoo! I see the magic number on the scale—that number is no longer controlling me, my actions, or my emotions. I am finally controlling it! Nothing gives my mind more freedom than that number on the scale. Goal weight, they call it.

A week or so passes and I have an argument with my boyfriend (or my mother or my father or my boss or my friend). I feel fat. I feel bored. Work is slow. I am sure all the other mothers at school are gossiping about ME. All my work colleagues are saying how I am this or that; my mother or my friend has just hinted at another diet for me to go on with them. Argh! I am feeling agitated, restless, irritable, and discontent.

Then a light bulb goes on and a voice tells me, "Some processed food will fix it. You have been so good—you can have some morning tea or a snack with your friends. Just one cupcake with sprinkles will be fine." Off I go and have it, and the experiment goes well. I stop after the second one. "Maybe I have been making too big a deal out of this," my thoughts tell me. I feel great and feel normal. I not only controlled my ingesting but enjoyed it too!!

Before I know it, lunchtime arrives, and a thought crosses my mind. "Why don't you get a takeaway for lunch, just a small serving, and even skip the apple pie. You have shown you can control *it now and you definitely won't binge." I feel fine, all is well. Next the negative voice reminds me, "It's the weekend—you don't need to exercise—your boyfriend (or my children or my job) needs you."*

But I think to myself, "I would like to go out to a smorgasbord for dinner. Nothing more." I make sure my husband (or my friend or my acquaintance) knows that I am only just going to eat an appetizer and a main dish. No dessert, but if I do, I ask them to remind me I'm only going to have one plateful of food for my dinner. I am so excited; I get to pile as much onto my plate as I want. I know I will be okay as I stopped after my breakfast this morning and my lunch too.

I go out to dinner and two hours later I find myself practically having to be dragged away, trying to make an excuse why I can now eat my third dessert, and wanting one more while convincing myself and everyone how OK it is, as on Monday I will go back on my diet ... so I might as well make the most of this now.

I binge plenty more that night, and then continue when I get home thanking my lucky stars my husband was so tired he went straight to bed. Then when I wake up the next day, I feel so guilty with this voice saying to me, "I told you to pull up after one meal. You should have listened to me. Now you are so fat you'll have to starve for the next week." My head starts to throb, my stomach aches, and I double over. It continues and says, "Why did you pick up* in the first place, you knew you would not be able to stop! You are such a failure, a failure at dieting, a failure at losing weight, in fact, a failure at life; you can't stick to anything." The guilt, remorse, self-pity, shame, and blame are indescribable. One more attempt and one more failure!

---

*Pickup is a term used in the addiction field for when a person experiences a slip or what is more commonly known as a relapse; that is, a person returns to ingesting processed food.

Miranda Shares

It is Sunday and I go to my friend's twenty-first birthday party. I have eaten very little for the last two days. I know now that one bite of processed foods won't hurt me. I have been so good, and I'm looking fantastic. "Loosen up," my mind whispers. "Jane would love you to be a party girl and enjoy her celebration with her. You have been a bit of a downer since you announced you were eliminating processed foods ... AND ... Jane reminded you that you only turn 21 (or 30 or 40 or 50) once!!! Yes, hmm, maybe Jane is right," I think. "I might just have a small sliver of the birthday cake—as they are cutting the cake early. I plan to have just one slice for now."

The voice is very encouraging. "You go, girl. Enjoy this, you deserve it, all right!" I am still hesitant. The disease voice knows this. "Go on. It won't hurt you this time—you are at your goal weight—and on Monday you can get back to the gym." I KNOW this time will be different, so I have a piece of cake. I look at the buffet table and hear another whisper. "You haven't had those types of processed food for ages. Some marinated chicken drumsticks, delicious! Fried rice, mmm! Little pastry parcels, some nuts, a handful of crackers and dip, and a slice of carrot cake."

My head starts to spin. The unnamed voice is now louder. "You had better eat all you can now as you will have to go on a diet tomorrow and I promise I will make sure you have the little bit of willpower you will need tomorrow, just trust in me."

My head is hurting as I return to the colored table with all the pretty foods calling to me and I try a little bit of everything, trying desperately to hide what I am doing and making infinite excuses why I am allowed to eat this tonight. I pull my waistband down underneath my bloated belly as it is starting to pinch. I feel very tired, but I can't stop. Before I know it, it is midnight, and everyone is leaving. The food counter is closed. What do I do now?

I fall asleep in the car and wake up at 2 a.m. at home in my own bed. I assume Jack must have helped me get into bed. I just need to go to the kitchen—frozen ice cream—that's Jack's—he won't mind. Frozen bread—better defrost it—but then everyone will hear the microwave go beep, beep, beep!!! Haven't they made a silent microwave YET!!! Not to worry—it will melt as I put some peanut butter, cheese, and banana on it, then put it under the griller.

After another feast, I go back up to bed, stomach aching.

I wake up at 9 a.m. the next morning. My head hurts even more. I feel disgusted with myself. Why did I have a piece of cake? I am now once again so fat. The disease voice is back. "Why did you have that piece of cake—you were doing fine until then. Now you're fat again." I panic and look in the mirror—my thighs are bigger than an elephant's; I get on the scales—I have put on 7 lb. (3 kg.) over the last three days. I definitely can't go to work today—I vow to start my diet right there and then. I have a moderate breakfast following the food plan diet's rules. I am feeling hopeful again.

Now it is 2 p.m. and my voice that seems to sit on my head dictating my every move with sweet promises to help me is back. "You might as well make the most of it now; a couple of days more won't hurt. Remember, you are owed a couple of sick days, plus you have ten days' sick leave left. And next Monday is your day off because of working a compressed work week, so you can start again then." This takes all the pressure off. Out come some laxatives to get me through the week and to push the food through. I watch movies on TV, mask my calls, and don't return any.

Do I vomit, purge, go to the gym for a couple of hours, exercise at home, go on a fast for a period of time? It is a constant battle to stop ingesting processed foods every day. Waiting, just waiting until Monday rolls around again. THIS TIME IT IS GOING TO BE DIFFERENT!

Joyce Shares

I am so disgusted with myself and so angry as to why I can't seem to keep my weight off. My thoughts are that my husband is going to tire of my ever-growing body soon. As long as he knows I'm trying, he probably won't confront me on it. Half of what I do to lose weight I know won't work. To be honest, that can be a plus on one hand, because when it does fail, I can keep on eating what I want, when I want, and as much as I want. That's what I want to do. I want to enjoy eating but control my eating. Why is that so hard??

I jump on the scale and it's not as bad as I thought. Since I have to live another day, I try to remember what I ate yesterday to get to this decent number. The scale says I'm okay, but I'm puzzled. I totally binged after dinner, only wanted a few cookies. If I didn't have an appetite, things would be different. I get hopeful.

My voice says, "Maybe you are getting more normal; keep cutting down just a bit more of what you eat, that's all you have to do. You will and can control this."

Yeah, I know. I got a whole lot of success with other things to prove to myself that if I try hard enough, I can do it. I can do it. I can do it, so why can't I just do it? I only need to be taught how.

I enter the next best program I've researched, motivated and feeling this time it will work. I can learn structure just like everyone else and then I will become a normal eater. Busting through the doors, I embrace the diet environment. I notice first how much and what kinds of food I can have. If there is literature to read, I will want the deluxe leather-bound versions to enhance my outcome. Tools and gadgets to get me to control myself by counting, selecting, journaling, tracking, and itemizing will be included in the bag.

My mind is set. I can eat all I want and as much as I want without consequences as long as it is okay with this program. The book says "6 ounces of fruit." "That's not enough," my inner voice says.

> "Half." Half of what? A cantaloupe! Don't they know cantaloupes come in all different sizes? I could get the biggest one I can find and have half of it. No one will know. Are they kidding? Suddenly, I become restless, irritable, and discontent.
>
> After a month or so, the scale shows fifteen pounds gone and I'm glad, but it's just not enough to override the dull way I've been feeling. I'm unhappy. I still want and obsess about eating processed food all the time. My resolution from one month ago faded since God knows when.
>
> "I can't fit this into my life anymore," I decide. I'll find some reliable excuse to drop out. They know I'm trying ... it just didn't work for me!!!

We each have a story to share. I would love to hear *your* story. If you would like to share your own story, I have a web page for you to post on. You may identify yourself or remain anonymous; you may share as little or as much as you would like. It is up to you. You are not alone anymore. Go to www.addictionology.com.au.

Processed Food Addict, Alcoholic, Drug Addict, Nicotine Addict, Codependent, Substance Abuser?

Could you identify with any of the sharing above? Individuals with a predisposition to ingest processed foods are unable to consume processed food without developing a phenomenon of craving—this is the common denominator. However, processed food addicts vary in the way they control it, eat it, get rid of it, hide it, and diet, to prove they will one day be able to eat like a normal eater. That is, to *control and enjoy* processed foods just like they see everyone else doing.

How then do I know that I may be succumbing to a malady known as *addiction*, or is it just in my imagination? Or perhaps I am a food abuser, and that means I'm making too big a deal out of it? Perhaps I had a dysfunctional upbringing? I feel I can be addicted to anything. Is that just my personality? Do I have one or multiple addictions?

Perhaps I could do a bit of coke to help burn off the calories from the last binge and to help control my depression. How many times have I put the smokes down then eventually gone back to smoking because it controls my weight for now? This is actually swapping the witch for the bitch (one substance for another) as I see fit.

Addiction is likened to cancer—meaning it is also a consumer of mind and body—and yet it is a very hidden, secretive disease. Indeed, it is often hidden under the disease of denial and the addicted person is usually the last one to find out. The acronym DENIAL (**D**on't **E**ven k**N**ow **I** **A**m **L**ying) says it all in a nutshell. Most people suffering from processed food addiction (PFA) are not **bad people trying to be good; they are just sick people trying to get well.**

Let's Share

> *My dream was to become an air hostess. I was eighteen, not quite old enough to apply for Qantas, so I applied for Ansett. These were the two airlines operating in Australia at that time. I was successful in my application; I made arrangements to fly interstate to train for my dream job. I was so excited as I was now at the airport waiting to catch my flight. I walked into a newsagent to get a book to read on the flight, and before I knew it I was taking a bite of a chocolate bar. Then, this phenomenon of craving kicked in, overriding any of my thoughts of catching a plane. I wanted to be an air hostess more than anything in the world, and yet I could not stop myself from ingesting more processed food. I did not make the flight, in fact I ended up in the airport's food court ingesting processed food in a way that was beyond my mental control.*

This confirms the eerie paradox of any addiction—the only way to feel better is to *use* the substance of choice, which in turn makes the addict feel worse. Hence, the problem. Processed foods (the substance) become the solution for many, thus keeping the merry-go-round of denial spinning!

What is a processed food addiction?

Processed food addiction is a fierce and tenacious disease, devilish in its means, unyielding in its onset, and corruptive and extensive in its effects on the body, mind, and soul. It is like a chameleon, as it manifests individually in many and varied stages as the disease progresses from one extreme to another. The extremes of the processed food addiction continuum are black and white, while the stages are the many shades of gray in between. It continues to be very subtle and elusive for clinicians and researchers to collegially and definitively arrive at a distinct definition, which at the best of times can be confusing and contradictory, depending upon one's biases and perspectives. Therefore, the language implemented to understand the disease of addiction—such as the diagnosis, prognosis and alternative treatment options—creates many and varied challenges. Adding to these challenges is how this information is portrayed to all levels of society including clinicians, patients, family members, work colleagues, policymakers, and the many and varied facets of media. For example, over the last two decades, there have been many definitions of the disease of addiction, which I have studiously followed and drawn upon. However, in originally defining processed food addiction, I too kept it as simple as possible to communicate a better understanding of the nature of the disease.

The Term "Processed Food Addiction"

In keeping things simple, especially when working with potential processed food addicts, I define processed food addiction simply:

> *An individual with processed food addiction cannot persistently anticipate, on any occasion when ingesting processed foods, the quantity that will be ingested or the duration of the binge.*
>
> (Raymond, 2016)

In April 2011, the American Society of Addiction Medicine (ASAM) issued a public policy statement regarding both a long and short definition of addiction, partly suggesting addiction is characterized by bio-psycho-social-spiritual manifestations.[2] However, this policy statement has now been archived and is no longer considered active ASAM policy.

As previously highlighted, the terminology in understanding today's diseases, and specifically addiction, continues to evolve. In 2019, ASAM redefined the definition of addiction to help clarify the meaning of addiction-related terms, as used by professional bodies. Analogous to 2011, ASAM (2019) redefined and adopted an updated definition of addiction stating.

> *Addiction is a treatable, chronic medical disease involving complex interactions among brain circuits, genetics, the environment, and an individual's life experiences. People with addiction use substances or engage in behaviors that become compulsive and often continue despite harmful consequences.*
>
> *Prevention efforts and treatment approaches for addiction are generally as successful as those for other chronic diseases.*
>
> *(Adopted by the ASAM Board of Directors, September 15, 2019)*

Likewise, as I continue to come to a greater and deeper understanding of the disease of processed food addiction in all its many and varied facets, I too have recognized and now acknowledge the need for an updated definition of processed food addiction. Hence, a twenty-first-century definition of processed food addiction would be more along these lines:

> *Processed food addiction is a treatable, chronic biochemical condition of the brain, coupled with a physiological condition of the body, linked to psychological, social, and spiritual manifestations.*
>
> *People with the disease of processed food addiction experience a mental obsession of the mind, coupled with a physiological powerlessness known as the phenomenon of craving; this in turn,*

> *makes the person continue to ingest processed foods no matter the circumstances.*
>
> (Raymond, 2019)

So, am I a processed food addict?

> *Call me a compulsive overeater, heavy eater, binge eater, emotional eater, anorexic, bulimic, food abuser, under-eater, psychologically dependent eater, recreational eater, impulsive eater, chocoholic—call me whatever you like, but please—oh please, please, please—don't call me a **processed food addict**!*

The word *addiction* typically suggests that the person who is an *addict*, a *junkie*, a *pill head*, an *alky*, or a *substance abuser* is out of control, has no willpower, or is basically doomed and should be locked up.

The labels and language used call up images of backyard drug labs with dudes abusing alcohol and getting high, and then causing bedlam in the neighborhood. This image gives a certain stigma to one suffering from the malady of addiction, with the added bonus of a common fallacy: "It is really about whether I have been good or bad." This thrusts the person into thinking they must have done something wrong to have "this thing," while spending infinite amounts of money to do better, fix it, and lose the stigma of addiction. Then we see the press come into play, painting an explicit narrative picture of what "the addict" did during the spree, followed by the addict expressing remorse and regret and promising to mend their ways.

Quite often I have a patient come into the clinic and share with me how they have tried everything to fix this thing. As with any chronic illness, a diabetic will never be able to think down their blood sugar, a cardiac patient will never run a marathon, and a real addict will never control and enjoy the substance in the way they see others doing at liberty. This is why diets, weight-loss rooms, exercise centers, gimmicks, and gyms (and the list rolls on endlessly) do not *work* for a processed food addict.

Does this excuse the potential addict for what they did while they were on their spree? Definitely not. However, if we can look at the addict as a sick person trying to get well rather than as a bad person trying to be good, we may make an inroad into a malady that seems to be destroying everything and everyone in its path while the person tries to fix something they cannot fix.

And no, not every person will want to get well. That is a topic for another time and well beyond the scope of what I am writing about for now.

Trillions of dollars are spent globally by people taking on the challenge to prove they can eat like a normal eater—that is, control and enjoy how much processed food one ingests while staying at goal weight. And I might add, goal weight changes over the years.

When faced with the probability of an addiction diagnosis, most people will try to tone down the label and call themselves *problem eaters* or *compulsive overeaters*. The term *food addict* may also be implied and can sit comfortably with the person, as so many people they know call themselves a *food addict* these days. "So, it can't be that bad," they reason. Of late, I have heard the term *junk food addict*. This label can still keep the real processed food addict in denial. Eliminating junk food is not as daunting or as severe as treating a disease of addiction. Meanwhile, they jump on the bandwagon, trying to prove they have the problem licked now, while they stick rigorously to different methods of control (diets, food plans, mindfulness courses, exercise regimes, control methods to keep the junk food down by not eating any takeout food), until one day they try the game again: just one little tiny morsel of "extra food," which leads to two morsels, to a slice, a bowl, a plate, and oblivion.

Let's Share

> *I seemed to be able to control my weight in the early days with this diet or that exercise, but as I got older and my bingeing progressed, I seemed to lose some of my willpower. I then had to go to a few more extreme measures. Laxative abuse (twenty tablets*

a night—ugh! All night on the toilet with blisters on my butt and horrific stomach cramps. Some deep cleansing also helped for a while, but I had this horrific never-ending desire to ingest some processed food in some way, shape, or form.

I ended up learning that I could be just a compulsive overeater. It sounded right, as I would be going great guns and then I would get this compulsion to eat that was so powerful, it was like a magnetic force to the fridge. I couldn't stay abstinent like the others in the group.

Then I learned if I followed a specific food plan, I would be okay.

Then that didn't work, so I heard the term food addict. *That was a better label and seemed to be okay, as everyone else seemed fine with it. I also had to implement a bit more control, that is, weigh and measure what I ate, and every now and again I could get away with a bit more of this or a bit more of that. No one had to know. I loved the get-togethers and the scientific knowledge telling me about my brain, and I loved the support, but a lot of them seemed to be doing really well but me. I once had over one-and-a-half years of abstinence, but then I ingested just a little bit and I couldn't stop. So, I changed from this person to that person. Sought more counselors, psychologists, psychiatrists, all sorts of health professionals. I even went to health resorts and places to help me eliminate the substance. We prayed and meditated each day; they knew what I could and could not eat. But then I would leave and sooner or later, I would ingest the processed food again.*

"What is wrong with me?" I pondered this question many, many, many times, especially seeing others appearing to have some measure of control, which for the life of me, I did not have. Paradoxically, at times I felt like I was finally getting back some control. BUT sooner or later, a thought to ingest would come out of the blue, or sometimes I wouldn't even think about it and boom, I was off again. It was so hard and exhausting to hide my binges from my family, friends, work colleagues, study buddies, and even the neighbors.

I am sure they have seen me take food out of my trash can that I put in the night before.

Is everyone a processed food addict?

Definitely not. Not everyone who ingests processed foods is a processed food addict! That is like saying everyone who drinks alcohol is an alcoholic.

I will give you an example. If a person continues to ingest processed foods and the consequences (which are those problems that keep accumulating, including weight gain, health issues, social rejection, and more) and their life *continue* to become more out of control, then odds are the person is a processed food addict. Paradoxically, for a particular period of time, it may not be apparent that the root cause of this crisis (of not being able to control weight gain, with anxiety, depression and stress becoming ever more present daily) is the ingestion of processed food. Some individuals learn this lesson faster, while others learn by doing it over and over again. However, a lifetime of weight watching, attending gyms, and trying methods to *control* and *enjoy* one's processed food intake certainly make one inclined to think that a processed food addict is in our midst.

Chapter Two

Questions, Questions, Questions

Why me?

"Why me?" is a good question people ask. Why is it that some people do not have an addictive reaction to processed foods and others are clearly compelled to face the fact that they will never be able to ingest processed foods again?

"Why me?" is the question I get asked most in my clinic, as misfortune after misfortune befalls the person sitting in front of me. They raise their face to the sky and ask, "Why me?" A rhetorical question, presumably between themselves and their deity. Of course, this question has also confused academics and social theorists trying to understand the baffling nature of the obvious physical and psychological symptoms of addiction.

What does "a sick brain" mean in the context of processed food addiction?

Fundamentally, the term *a sick brain* means that a processed food addict needs the substance—processed foods—to be able to function; hence, the brain is *hijacked* by the processed foods and the person is under their influence. This brings up the topic of tolerance, which is part of the addiction: an addict develops a tolerance for processed foods and forms a dependency on it. Tolerance manifests as a reduction in sensitivity to a substance (Herron & Brennan, 2015). Significant changes in cellular structure occur that allow the body to function normally even when ingesting copious amounts of processed foods.

In the early stages of processed food addiction, a processed food addict is mostly impaired *not* when they ingest processed foods but when they stop ingesting the processed foods. Usually, they have learned to keep a bag of chips or candies or a nut bar in their work drawer, briefcase, or glove box, "just in case" the all-too-familiar withdrawal syndrome kicks in. These emergency supplies of processed foods allow the addict to function normally and to put off the withdrawal symptoms, such as headaches and feeling mentally confused, which can be so excruciating and incapacitating.

The torturous pain of withdrawal is so horrific that an addicted person will go to any lengths to make sure they don't have to endure it while among others. Hence secretive, sneaky, and crafty behaviors come into play, such as endless trips to the restroom. What's really happening is the processed food addict (unbeknown to them) is protecting themselves (temporarily) against the physical, mental, and spiritual suffering of withdrawal.

A processed food addict will justify and rationalize psychological symptomology as a means of excusing their ingestion of processed foods. "I eat because I am breastfeeding." "My husband is away at the moment." "My job is becoming quite stressful."

The processed food addict believes they can defuse their restlessness, irritability, and discontent only by ingesting the processed foods again. Thus, the processed food addict's brain is a sick brain. The only rational cognitive thought the brain can understand is that it needs and demands the processed food if it is to function at all. And as for the processed food addict, they consciously and subliminally know that enduring withdrawal is a nightmare compared to succumbing to the processed foods again, as so many do.

I will go into tolerance and withdrawal symptoms a bit more in depth later.

Let's Share

I always have a packet of candies and some nuts in my drawer at work. I just pop one in my mouth to stay awake and be able to do my work until I can get out to the staff room at lunchtime.

I have gum everywhere, in my drawer at work, in the car glove box, in my bedside drawer, because when I chew, it helps me feel like I can control my processed food intake and at the same time makes me feel better, or at least until I can get my hands on something that will kick in so much quicker, like some dried fruit or the cookies in the staff room.

If my weight is normal, how could I possibly be a processed food addict?

Some people who are predisposed to processed food addiction have used a myriad of methods to stay in denial while aspiring to control their weight and look normal or healthy. Some of these methods include excessive exercise; vomiting; laxative abuse; daily, weekly, or biweekly detoxes; cleanses; fasting; smoking; going on long hikes; using a professional sport status to control the substance; jaw wiring; staying at health retreats; and weight-loss surgery. All of this is done to eliminate a major life-threatening symptom of processed food addiction, which is overweight. I have only mentioned a few methods. However, if one is a processed food addict, the control becomes harder and harder due to an increase in one's tolerance to processed food. *Tolerance* means the need or desire or craving to ingest more and more processed foods—for example, three-quarters of a large pizza, instead of two or three slices, with garlic bread; or at least half a packet of chocolate cookies and two bottles of coke; or a box of cereal with chocolate milk, plus four slices of cinnamon toast with heaps of butter on white bread—to get the same effect as before. Simultaneously, withdrawal symptomology increases such symptoms as, for example, depression; anxiety and stress; feelings of worthlessness, anger, and hopelessness; and the notion that one is down for the count.

Olivia Shares

> I have had a few problems with my weight over the years, but I have weighed 132 lb. (60 kg.) for the past three years. Although over the past decade I might have gone up only about 6.6 lb. (3 kg.), not enough for anyone to notice, the truth is that I just starve myself and get it back down again or increase my gym sessions. I find, though, that the starving and/or dieting is getting harder to do, and the gym is repetitious and boring at times. So to get me back on track, I have now started to include detoxes every second week, and when I can afford it, I save up to go to a health retreat to eliminate the junk food—foods which I have identified as problem foods and trigger foods. I find laxatives are a good backup too because I feel at least I'm doing something to justify that I'm uncontrollably ingesting processed foods.
>
> BUT my head won't stop punishing me for ingesting the processed foods, rhetorically telling me, "I've busted from my diet and I'm now going to be morbidly obese. I'm losing control. Don't tell anyone because they will think I'm 'bad.' If I don't lose more weight, I will be unlovable." So, I continue to struggle. I just wish I could tell someone what is really going on, but my head says, "You can't tell anyone about this; they won't believe you."

This potential processed food addict stays in denial with the adage that because she is not overweight, she could not possibly be a processed food addict.

Angela Shares

Angela shares that she was diagnosed with an eating disorder, got help, and now seems to be doing okay. However, in the last five or so years, the disorder has started to "come back again," and it seems to have gotten worse.

> *In the past, I could get away with some processed foods and be fine, but now even ingesting something that isn't on my diet plan creates this desire to want more, and then this uncontrollable craving for more kicks in. I feel like I am losing control and I'm so scared.*

Just because a person may have been diagnosed with an eating disorder, this does not give them immunity to having processed food addiction.

I must clarify here that there are some people who are able to control their eating disorder if they have an adequate mental analysis and a sufficiently strong reason to do so. For example, they have found the person of their dreams; they are moving internationally for a fantastic job opportunity; the doctor says they will die if they don't get well now; they get pregnant, or their wife or partner has a baby, and they believe they have something to live for. This may give the person the much-needed motivation to moderate or significantly cut down their processed food consumption. Medical interventions may also become operational here; even though the person may find it problematic to cut down on their own, with medical intervention they find they are able to either moderate, control, or stop ingesting processed food.

Let's Share

Joan has been up and down with her weight for the past thirty years. She put on approximately 20–30 lb. (9–14 kg.) and then went to a weight-loss center to try and lose it. But then she found she needed more help to keep it under control, so she joined an anonymous food group and found a spiritual way of life. The support and identification each week helped her get by, accepting that she puts some on but she can also take it off, especially if she has a reason to do so.

Is Joan a processed food addict? Who is to say? Many people abuse addictive substances and they are quite happy most days getting by, and may do so until they are in their later years.

On the Other Hand ...

Janine shares that she was obese for the first fifty-plus years of her life, so she sought help and got weight-loss surgery. Janine lost approximately 99 lb. (40 kg.) over a period of eighteen months, got surgery to tighten the loose skin, and was feeling normal for the first time in her life. However, two and a half years later, she believed her relationships seemed to be confusing and thwarted; her job wasn't as exciting and was going downhill; her stepchildren seemed to want more and more of her time; and her husband wouldn't stop nagging.

> *At first, I knew I couldn't eat after the surgery like I used to, but I found I could get away with a cup of coffee and a muffin, or suck melted chocolate through a straw. This helped me to cope with life, and even alcohol seemed to be okay, in small amounts, of course. It made me feel so much better. Took away all my problems ... at least for a while.*

As I mentioned earlier, alcohol is produced by the natural fermentation of sugars. So, the morbidly obese person is still ingesting processed food, but in liquid form, sparking off the phenomenon of craving.

Because she had the surgery, Janine is fighting against herself *not* to give in to the craving. Then the mental wars may start, with a negative voice whispering sweet nothings in her ears: "You have to stay in control; you paid so much to have this done. What will your family and friends say if they see you eating out of control?" Or "Just keep drinking some wine; it won't hurt you. Your operation was for being overweight; wine won't put on weight and you can control it."

Or the whisperings can do what I call a flip. "It's been eighteen months now since the operation. You deserve to have just a little bit of extra ice cream, that's all."

Generally, the potential processed food addict will have infinite ways to self-justify why they do this and why they do that. I often say, "An addict can convince anybody of anything." For example, they can convince those around them that how much the addict ingests, drinks, or uses is their fault. Sadly, the potential processed food addict is in denial and does not have a clue, or doesn't even know they are lying. Repetition is the mother of wisdom: remember, the acronym DENIAL stands for "Don't Even Know I Am Lying."

In treating processed food addiction, the saying goes "If someone has had weight-loss surgery, they have two years to get their sh*t together." Said in another way, even though the weight (symptom) has dissipated, the processed food addiction (cause) is still operational. Unfortunately, some of the medical and health professions appear to not understand the real problem, or more to the point, do not take it seriously enough to change. And quite often these professionals will never get to the truth about the extent of the disease in the potential processed food addict. Once again I reiterate, processed food addiction is a ferocious, relentless illness. It is diabolical in its means, subtle and deceptive in its onset, fiendish in its effects on the body, and a seducer of mind, body, and spirit, while it continues on a rampage throughout the world.

Janice Shares

> *After topping off the scale at 302, reflecting a hundred-plus-pound (45-kg.) weight gain from quitting smoking, I broke both feet only eight weeks apart and had to give up my job as an active ER nurse. I tried one more program, this time a group hypnosis with 175 people in a ballroom, which worked just until I got out to the parking lot.*
>
> *After this one, I was going for bariatric surgery. It was going to be risky for sure, but the means to an ultimate end.*
>
> *The doctor informed me I was not to eat sugar, as it would ruin the weight-loss outcome. In total denial, I assured him that would not*

be a problem, that I only liked pasta, pizza, and chips, that sugar was not my problem, and I believed it.

Little did I know that the cravings, desire, and obsession for food, more processed food, after surgery would be exactly the same as before. The only change was that I could no longer volumize (overeat on any food) without becoming sick. I continued to push the limits of my stomach capacity, always by mistake.

During the two-year process of rapid expected weight loss, I began to entertain both patients and staff on my unit by purchasing and serving food for parties. Monthly, for thirty people, I'd buy eight extra-large pizzas, 125 chicken wings, side orders, six liters of soda, desserts, candy, and all the paper goods. I would stand there and watch everyone else eat, vicariously engaging my hijacked brain to experience something I still needed, as others ingested all the food I wanted. These parties continued for over a year, all at my expense.

Another nurse at work told me many times about a casino she went to and all the money that she had won there. I eventually went and took my elderly father with me. Winning only a hundred dollars that night, I successfully switched the witch for the bitch. I believe this one thrill—that first time—turned into a sixteen-year serious and progressive gambling addiction. I actually began to use my long hours of compulsive gambling as a way to manage my desire to eat processed foods as well. Eventually, half of the five-year weight loss came back on and I knew I had to start dieting again or else, only now I had both problems.

The processed food addict in general leads a double life. On one hand, they will portray to the world that everything is okay: they are successful in business, responsible family members, socially active, and a jolly good person overall, dependable and reliable. Or maybe they acknowledge they have "a bit of a food issue, but it is under control" because they are still functioning (albeit at an increasingly limited capacity as the disease continues to progress).

On the other hand, let them indulge in some processed foods for a while and they will become unreliable, irresponsible, forgetful, and full of denial. Within themselves, they will be deeply regretful as they remember what they did over the period of the last splurge, hoping that no one saw them. These memories are then buried deep down inside them, and they hope against hope that no one will be on to them and expose their secret. Being under such pressure 24-7, of course, brings about more bingeing. Very rarely will a processed food addict tell those in the medical field the whole truth, or if they do, it will be justified by "I am so depressed, full of anxiety and fearful (and so on, for the rationalizing), which is why I do it."

If the professional presents a solution (the latest healthy diet, a dietitian's number, or something else), very seldom will the patient follow any of the instructions and guidance given. It is little wonder then that some medical professions have a low opinion of the processed food addicts (disguised under many labels) who continually come to them time and time again asking for help but going away and doing exactly what they did in the past, only now they are worse than the last time. Secondary symptoms (the primary symptom being processed food addiction), including hypertension, preliminary signs of heart disease, type 2 diabetes, and prediabetes diagnoses, continue to arise and may spiral out of control.

Processed food addiction appears to be one of the basic roots of disorders that the medical profession perceives as primary diseases, like obesity, diabetes, hypertension, and cardiac disease. Typically, the medical professional does not look at processed food addiction. Instead, they treat the secondary disease process stemming from processed food addiction. What the potential processed food addicts are ingesting is overlooked while the health-care practitioner is laboriously working on the secondary illnesses and symptoms.

This approach is similar to when a patient presents with symptoms of, for instance, type 2 diabetes or pneumonia. The clinician does not treat the high blood sugar or the high temperature but sends the patient home, saying, "Now that your blood sugar or high temperature has subsided, keep an eye on that diabetes or pneumonia."

Unfortunately, this appears to be what's happening globally with processed food addiction. The clinician may take care of the symptoms of the secondary diseases by saying to the patient, "Now that your essential symptoms have dissipated (your temperature, blood pressure, blood sugar levels), don't eat too much takeout."

I Thought I Was ...

> My family helped me to see a professional for my many ailments. It has been approximately four-plus years. I feel hopeful I'm getting better, but I seem to be getting worse.

This is as good a time as any to share about the enabler, which is one of many roles others may play in a potential processed food addict's life. *Enabling* is about creating patterns that continue to operate within networks of families, friends, work colleagues, and communities (e.g., church groups or weight-loss groups) that may keep a person addicted to their substance by "rescuing" them. Typically, these dysfunctional associations allow the addicted individual to avoid taking responsibility and facing the full consequences of their addiction. Justification, ignoring the problem, denying, or even excusing the addict can smooth over the addiction, time and time again.

> A professional person may also be an enabler (a person in the church, lawyer, doctor, addiction counselor, social worker, etc.). This can be potentially quite damaging, as it may condition those involved with the person to curtail the crisis instead of initiating a treatment program to bring about their recovery. As the processed food addiction and its trail start to spread outside the family unit, the individual generally seeks help from a professional, who may not be adequately qualified to deal with addiction. This then

secures a reduction of their dilemma by using the professional as an enabler, making them responsible for fixing the situation, so the addict can get back to doing and enacting the only life they know— that is, proving to the world and mostly themselves that they are normal when it comes to controlling processed foods.

I have learned that if I can control my behavior and thinking around processed food, over time I will not want it. I have also learned that I have a malfunction in my brain, so now that I know what is wrong with me, I won't need to ingest processed food again, or better still, someday I will be able to control and enjoy eating processed food in a normal way, just like everyone else, now that I know what is wrong with me.

Unfortunately, this continues to keep not only the processed food addict in denial, but also everyone involved with the processed food addict. The roundabout of denial for both the enablers and the processed food addict spins around and around, getting nowhere. Meanwhile, the illusion that the processed food addict is trying hard continues, breeding more self-pity while also keeping the delusion alive that in the past they *had* been able to control their intake of processed foods. This then elevates the obsession that "one day, just like I did two (or five or ten) years ago, I will be able to control *and* enjoy eating processed foods—I will be normal."

The potential processed food addict tries and works on her behaviors, plus she changes her thinking. Meanwhile, she does not know that addiction is a progressive disease. Over time, it gets worse, never better, if one is a "real" processed food addict.

Indeed, factors including psychological, social, financial, environmental, and/or ethnicity do influence the advancement of processed food addiction. As the addiction literature posits, they do have a part to play. However, for a person to start ingesting processed foods addictively, the person must by some means be physiologically able to accept large amounts of processed foods into their system, which is essential in keeping the addiction operational. Unless the person has the physical susceptibility to become addicted, they will be able to control and enjoy their eating. People who are not processed food addicts (non-PFAs) do not experience this phenomenon of craving; they do not need to ingest greater and greater amounts of processed foods, spend hours (days, months, or years) looking for new methods to control their weight, and in turn, do not experience increased withdrawal symptoms as they continue to ingest processed foods. What's more, for the non-PFA, it is a much easier choice to stop ingesting processed foods when they have had enough; it is a more excruciating choice for a real processed food addict. In other words, it is comfortable for a non-PFA to stop ingesting processed foods but a more torturous choice for the processed food addict to do the same.

Jenny Shares

> *I know I am overweight, but I don't think I have a problem with it. I have finally accepted this is the way I am, so why does everyone judge me? Of course, deep down I would like to be thinner, but hey, my friends are also obese—even bigger than me. Life would be not worth living if I couldn't go out with my friends and eat what they are eating.*

This may also be true for a lot of people who are overweight or obese. However, it can be a form of denial for those with a predisposition to processed food addiction.

Dianna Shares

> *I am confused about processed food addiction. I don't binge eat often. I drink Coke to help me to stay sober and I eat a few candies, cakes, and snacks and drink the coffee at my Alcoholics Anonymous meeting. After AA, we might go out to a takeaway, normally a pizza joint or fish and chips. I recently tried to give up smoking, but every time I do, I put on weight. Instantly, my anxiety and*

stress levels go through the roof. I got some medications to help me sleep and take care of my anxiety, and the clinician suggested I go to Overeaters Anonymous. Some days are better than others, though. I am sure it is my psychological problems that are causing my weight gain. My mother smoked until she was well into her eighties. I'm sober, that's all that matters.

When I met Di, I could see from her physical appearance that her weight was well over 275 lb. (125 kg.) and rising, and yet in Di's mind, her psychological problems were causing her weight gain. Thus she was taking medications to help with her psychological instability. She rationalized that "like her mother," she too, could keep smoking.

Perhaps Di can, and perhaps Di cannot.

In reality, these psychological symptoms are secondary to the disease of processed food addiction. If Di is a processed food addict, the Coke, coffee, medications, nicotine, and anything else that is used to control any symptomology of PFA (and keep Di in denial) will not be able to control it forever. What is so mesmerizing to most people is that this person is morbidly obese with several other complications and yet in her mind she is still okay.

There is a difference between a person who is not addicted to processed foods (a non-PFA) and a person who is severely addicted to processed foods. Most people (that is, non-PFAs), when faced with the choice of either (1) getting help or (2) trying to live as best they can with a potentially fatal disease, will opt for getting help without a second thought.

But the real processed food addict, faced with the same choice, will spend quite a lot of time weighing up the options: "Shall I live the way I am, trying to blot out the reality of the situation as best I can, and eventually face the secondary complications that include diabetes, cardiac disease, hypertension, cancer, and death, or shall I seek help?" It seems that some people will change their religion, gender, environment, country—anything—rather than accept the reality of having a processed food addiction, even in the face of dire consequences.

At 287 lb. (130 kg.) Henrietta has been trying to diet as long as she can remember. She has tried all types of weight-loss methods, but the only relief she has is to keep on going back to the processed foods.

> *I just can't help it. I know I'm so overweight, but who cares? So I just have to live with it, but it is getting worse.*

This person is imprisoned in her body. When she looks in the mirror, she says, "I only *ever* look from the neck up or the ankles down." Once again, this type of PFA does not realize in all honesty the extent of the seriousness of her obesity, and therefore can come up with a million excuses under the sun to justify why this or why that!

Aprocessed food addict can be normal weight (145 lb., or 66 kg.), overweight (220+ lb., or 100+ kg), or underweight (99 lb., or 45 kg.), depending of course on particular personal characteristics such as height, gender, and country. Weight is the symptom; the disease of processed food addiction is the problem. All processed food addicts have one thing in common—they cannot start ingesting processed foods without developing the phenomenon of craving.

I Know I'm Different

> *I have tried to give up the junk food and the sugar, flour, and wheat, but I keep going back sooner or later. I start with nuts and dried fruit, that's all!*

> *I feel like someone who tries over and over to quit drinking, but I can't. Why not?*

With an addiction, there is no easier or softer way. Ask any recovered addict who has come out the other side. The only way out is to go through the recovery process. All we need is a little bit of *hope*—the willingness to take a peek, let our guard down ever so slightly and see what is on the other side of the fence. This is the beginning of the change that keeps hope alive.

> *I just had an argument with my partner who says food is different from what he calls a real addiction. everyone knows what an alcoholic or a drug addict is, but a processed food addict? Perhaps he is right.*

In 1994 I had the pleasure of working with a professor in the US who was involved with individuals attending the 12 step fellowship of Overeaters Anonymous. I said to him, "Processed food addiction is different from alcoholism or a drug addiction: we must eat every day. An alcoholic or a drug addict can eliminate the alcohol, nicotine, or even the drugs."

With a wry smile, as I am sure he had heard this remark many times before, the professor replied, "Same disease, different substance." He continued,

> *An alcoholic still has to drink every day (water, soft drinks, tea, milk, juice, etc.); they just do not under any circumstance drink anything with alcohol—they eliminate alcohol. A nicotine addict still has to breathe fresh air every day for survival. They breathe in clean air (oxygen) and they just don't inhale any nicotine whatsoever—they eliminate nicotine. A gambler still uses money in his daily life, but he stops gambling. And a processed food addict has to eat every day for survival (protein, carbohydrates, fruit, vegetables, oil, dairy). They eliminate processed foods, that is, they only eat dairy, fruit, vegetables, salads, whole rice, and legumes, one day at a time.*

Nowadays, since so many oils have undergone so much processing, I would exchange his *oils* for *good fats*. For health, I recommend polyunsaturated oils: one serving per day for women and two servings per day for men. (Please see chapter 7 for more in-depth information.)

The professor's explanation gave me a greater understanding of the disease of addiction, while clearing up all the confusion that I seemed to be irrationally plagued with day and night.

How can food be addictive when it is a natural substance?

Especially when I see everyone else ingesting processed food with impunity. Globally, the top recreational drugs vary from leafy debris smoked in papers to pills. They have been processed from their raw form through the practices of distillation, crystallization, and concentration. Cocaine is a typical example, with its original state being coca leaves. It can be infused in liquid, processed into powder for nasal inhalation (snorting, sniffing), injected, ingested, or even used as a suppository. The result of this processing is what affects the neurological pathways in the brain.

Similarly, processed foods are refined and processed until they are no longer in their natural state.

The alcoholic is unable to drink alcohol without experiencing the phenomenon of craving. The same is true for the processed food addict. They cannot ingest processed foods in any way, shape, or form without sparking off the phenomenon of craving.

> *I prefer to eat alone; I feel everyone is judging me.*
>
> *AND... I hate how I must keep hiding what, where, and how much I eat from everyone. It is so exhausting.*

There are various reasons why processed food addicts like to eat in isolation. (In fact, I have found isolation and addiction go hand in hand.) Usually they do not want anyone to know how much they eat or to see the way they eat. Thus, it is quite typical for a processed food addict to stuff down several cookies or crackers or chocolates *before* attending a party where they know there will be a buffet of processed foods available. Usually, the processed food addict knows they will not get enough to fill their needs if they leave it to chance. This is why a processed food addict must stuff her purse, her pockets, or her partner's pockets with extra processed food. Such addicts have also been found in the washroom eating extra processed food from the array of party foods, which they stuffed in their bra or purse, or wrapped in napkins. Meanwhile, the host is forever refilling the banquet.

Most processed food addicts share if they get caught in the act. They usually feel so humiliated that they compensate by having an abundant supply of well-practiced speeches of self-justification and rationalization: "I'm hormonal at the moment, so I'm craving some sugar." "I've been so busy working that I missed breakfast and only had a snack at lunchtime." "I'm at goal weight now, and I allow myself one day a week when I can eat what I want." "I've just found out I'm pregnant." "This extra food isn't for me, it's for my husband (or dog or friend)." "I'm getting weight-loss surgery, so I'm having one last binge before I prepare for that."

A processed food addict is intrinsically ashamed and embarrassed of the way they ingest processed foods, no matter how much they may brazenly insist they are just having fun. In reality, the processed food addict doesn't know why they can't stop of their own accord. Not knowing they are addicted to processed foods (or even having some inkling but still trying to use willpower), they believe they are forlorn, inconsolable, and weak. There is always one more attempt and one more failure at trying to stop ingesting processed food, or at the very least cut down their consumption. Of course, once again this feeds shame, embarrassment, and guilt. They make countless excuses, some plausible, some not, especially in light of the horrific consequences that follow. If you are perhaps a processed food addict reading this, I'm sure you can add quite a few of your own excuses. What's even more alarming is that the processed food addict may appear stubborn, obstinate, arrogant, and/or headstrong. Their addiction is actually devising actions they may take, and in turn, overrides their ability to make rational and mentally sound decisions.

I am good all day but find I have to get up through the night and eat. Why?

Night-eating syndrome (NES) may be another symptom of a processed food addiction. Usually, this class of processed food addict will *graze* through the day ("being good," they call it), but after not eating much throughout the day, they crave a bite of processed food. More importantly, they need the processed foods to thwart the onset of the well-known torture of withdrawals. The processed food addict's body chemistry is out of whack. Over the years, their brains have become adapted to the presence of large amounts of processed foods in their system, which is used as the energy source for them to function.

In the severe stages of alcoholism, upon waking up in the morning, an alcoholic will hold a cup in their trembling hands with difficulty. Once the alcoholic has consumed some alcohol, they are better able to hold the cup without spilling the liquid. The same happens with a severe processed food addict. That first bite of processed food is needed to get back to what has become normal for them if they are to function at all. However, this form of processed food addiction happens mostly during the night. The brain does not care whether it is day or night, so long as it gets the hit—which keeps the individual in denial. They might say, "I've been good all day, so I deserve this," or "If I ingest processed food at night, it won't be anywhere near as bad as what I would have ingested in the daylight hours."

Self-knowledge avails us nothing. Why?

> I have read a fair bit about addiction, attended self-help groups as suggested, and spoken with a counselor at work, and now I know with all my heart I should not ingest processed foods, and yet I still do. ARGH!

In the addiction field, "self-knowledge avails *me* nothing" for a real processed food addict.

Over the last two decades, numerous studies in the bio-psycho-social-spiritual realms of addiction have investigated similarities between alcoholism, drug addiction, and food addiction. However, even when a processed food addict devours this literature (an addict is always trying to work out why she is addicted, and then she will go to great extremes to fix it) and understands she has a bio-psycho-social-spiritual underpinning that influences her to keep on using, she still turns around and ingests, drinks, and uses again. This is the puzzling feature of addiction.

Today I find more and more that I don't hone in on this methodology or that methodology but keep my eyes on results. What seems to be working long term when it comes to treating processed food addiction? How does the processed food addict keep the disease in remission (with peace of mind), similarly to other substance abusers?

After many years of receiving addiction treatments, my patients are what I call the professionals when it comes to the diagnosis, treatment, and relapse prevention of processed food addiction. I have been able to take their experiences into the research arena. They continue to teach me more and more each day in the clinic about the cunning, baffling, and powerful nature of this bizarre disease.

Why do I keep going back to eat again when I don't want to?

Let's look at the thinking that controls a processed food addict who repeats over and over again the frantic experiment of ingesting that first bite of processed food. After all the heartbreak and hardship they have gone through—dysfunctional relationships; psychological distress; emotional emptiness; becoming jobless, more often than not; feelings of despair, worthlessness, hopelessness, and uselessness; unhappiness and fear; lack of real purpose in life—why then do they still go into a bakery? What on earth are they thinking?

Josephine has been with her husband for over fifteen years—they were childhood sweethearts, have two children, and live in the suburbs of Brisbane. Josephine owns her own thriving hairdressing and beauty salon, which she has built up over the last decade. She has a charismatic personality; everyone loves her. She is an exceptional hairdresser, excelling in color and cuts.

Josephine's body type was slim, accompanied with an air of grace. She kept her figure trim by going to the gym every morning before starting work. She rarely ingested processed foods, until her first pregnancy at thirty. Over the next couple of years, she attended weight-loss programs to control her unhealthy eating. Then she used diet pills to give her enough energy to go to work and to be a wife and a mother. Then came the laxatives and visits to health resorts "to get my body back in shape." In just a couple of years, she started attending intensive psychological therapy; as she said, "I think I am losing my mind." She ended up selling her salon to her manager, who was delighted to take it on. After her last stint of bingeing, with one more attempt and one more failure, Josephine was given my contact details.

I shared with Josephine about the disease of processed food addiction being an illness that consumes mind and body. She spoke with and listened to other recovered processed food addicts and commenced to implement a prescribed stringent program and to encompass a spiritual way of life, as others were doing as though their lives depended on this process. Josephine started to prosper, returning to work three days a week. Her family life was restored to some semblance of functionality; however, she started tampering with her treatment program. Nothing happened in the beginning, but soon Josephine started disregarding the guides given to her and eventually she relapsed. Josephine was bewildered, finding herself bingeing and purging through exercise, laxatives, body cleansings, and detoxes.

Several times while working with Josephine, I shared that she was suffering from the malady of addiction. She knew she had a problem every time she ingested processed foods and that she had to do something about it long term or, she said, "I will go insane." And yet she binged again.

Josephine Shares

Here is Josephine's account of what happened.

> *I had a lovely weekend with the kids and was a bit tired on Sunday night, so I decided I would go for a drive to the beach. I thought a*

walk in the fresh air would do me good. My husband said he would drop off the kids at school and pick them up. I often went to Mooloolaba Beach just to clear my mind, taking my processed-food-free lunch with me.

The fresh air in my lungs and the sea breeze invigorated me. I sat down to have my abstinent lunch (4 oz of chicken, 6 oz of rice, 8 oz raw vegetables, 1 tbsp. of oil). Many times over the last twelve months I have sat on the beach and enjoyed my lunch.

All around me on the beach, families were enjoying burgers and french fries. I had no thought of ingesting processed foods. I realized I'd forgot my water, so I went to the shop and bought a bottle of water. No thought of ingesting processed foods. I then picked up a couple of napkins. Still no thought of ingesting.

Out of the blue, I was struck by the thought that I could order some french fries to go with my meal. It would be fine, as I could count them as my carb instead of the rice; so, I ordered some fries. Even though this did not feel right, I felt confident I could include the fries as my carbohydrate intake for the meal. I remembered my friend said I would have to start stabilizing my weight now anyway, so I wouldn't lose any more. This would help—that I was sure. I enjoyed those fries so much, and all seemed to be fine. So I got some more, with some extra gravy.

Josephine sparked off the allergy, the phenomenon of craving, by believing she could ingest the fries and include them in her meal without any consequences. She *knew* why she could not ingest processed foods in any way, shape, or form. She had been over and over it with her treatment team, mentor, sponsor, recovery buddies, and spiritual advisor, and yet all logic went out the window when the irrational thought kicked in to have fries with her lunch.

This is what is plainly called insanity. Doing the same thing over and over again and expecting a different result. This is what has baffled health professionals for decades. How on earth did Josephine not realize that one crumb of processed food would lead her to her "own hell on earth," as she described it.

I think the most baffling feature of this malady is that the majority of people in our society *can* have a choice: some can abuse it and still be okay. But for a person with an addiction, the power of choice is withdrawn when it comes to whether they can ingest the substance or not.

It is like jumping back into a stormy sea that you have just been rescued from. The addicted person seems to have *no* protection system to *not* jump back into the sea. This is the baffling feature of addiction: an outright inability not to do it again. The processed food addict casually thinks or says, "It will be fine. One won't hurt me, I'll show you." Or doesn't even think of the consequences before ingesting processed foods. Then she wonders, "How on earth did I do this again?," with the next thought being, "I might as well binge for the rest of the weekend and I'll start my diet on Monday."

Why do I seem to be on this roundabout of deception?

I have come to observe over and over again that there is one surefire symptom of processed food addiction, and that is addicts lying about how much processed food they are ingesting. The lie to me is the first indicator something is not quite right. In reality, do normal eaters (non-PFAs) do that? Have to lie about what they eat? It is obvious that non-PFAs do not have to cover up their ingestion of processed foods, or the eating behaviors and attitudes that go with it, and they don't feel guilty for eating them. Conversely, the processed food addict lies primarily to themself and then to those around them.

Let's have a look at this scenario for a minute. I might get into an elevator with Jenny (a processed food addict) and Sally (a so-called normal eater, or non-PFA), who is eating a bar of chocolate at 9:00 a.m. I might say to Sally, "Hey, Sally, I saw you at McDonald's for breakfast and you're now having some chocolate?"

"Yep, K-L," she says. "I just came from a morning work meeting held at McDonald's, and afterwards a couple of colleagues stayed and helped me plan my fiancé's birthday party."

Sally has no reason to lie. She definitely feels no guilt, shame, or concern.

However, when I see Jenny in the same elevator eating a chocolate bar and I say to her that I saw her at McDonald's in the morning and jokingly add, "The golden arches didn't cut it, right?," there will be a problem. Automatically, Jenny will feel anxious, guilty, and more, and she will go to any lengths to give me umpteen excuses why she was at McDonald's and is now eating chocolate!

What is even more interesting is that no matter what we learn about the disease of processed food addiction, even those who are genuine processed food addicts will still try to show that they have been misunderstood and hence most definitely are not processed food addicts! All the while, they wait, hoping for the day they will be able to control *and* enjoy ingesting processed foods like everyone else.

There are trillions of ways a processed food addict tries to prove they are like normal eaters, including the following:

- eating just three moderate meals a day with nothing in between
- becoming a vegetarian
- eating only natural foods
- taking an oath not to ingest processed foods ever again
- going on health retreats
- swearing on the Bible
- committing to a personal trainer or sponsor or mentor to not eat sugar, flour, or wheat
- tracking how many calories have been consumed each day and not exceeding the limit
- buying the latest inspirational books and/or books on well-being

- attending weight-loss programs
- having someone else cook and deliver sugar-free low-carb meals
- studying for some kind of nutrition degree or taking up a vocational course to help understand all about dieting and nutrition
- enrolling in a psychology degree or a medical degree
- willingly going into rehabilitation to help sort everything out
- getting tested for other maladies, such as diabetes, and hoping against hope that there is something else wrong and this was all a dream.

A *real* processed food addict has infinite reasons to prove they are different, which of course keeps them in denial for much longer. We have seen it repeat over and over again: someone who is a real processed food addict will one hundred percent not be able to stop ingesting processed food on a foundation of self-knowledge. There is no simpler solution than to eliminate processed foods and then seek the appropriate addiction treatment. Once a processed food addict, always a processed food addict!

My doctor tells me I must get the weight off. Why can't I keep it off?

> I know I am sick, and I hate myself. My doctor says if I don't lose the weight, I am in danger of putting my life at risk, or at the least my life span will be shortened, but I still can't stop ingesting processed foods.

Ingesting processed foods in spite of being overweight or obese, feeling psychologically distressed every time they are ingesting, having relationship problems, and having other physical illnesses, such as diabetes, hypertension, or heart disease, for example, are still not enough symptoms to dissuade a processed food addict from ingesting processed foods. The effect that comes from that first bite of processed food is so deceptive that, despite ominous warnings, the processed food addict can't tell what is real and what is make-believe: to them, ingesting processed foods is the norm.

This is a baffling feature of processed food addiction.

As the processed food addict is psychologically distressed—anxious, depressed, and having irrational thoughts and fears, with an underlying desire to ingest that first succulent bite of processed food for its accompanying feeling of contentment and calm—they will eventually give in to temptation. This is the norm for a practicing processed food addict. Once again, the phenomenon of craving develops, and before they know it they are in the familiar stage of bingeing. After the splurge, their thoughts turn to self-pity and repentance, which they then turn to making the next plan of *never* ingesting processed foods again.

One processed food addict described the phenomenon of craving as like having a wound that won't heal or an itch that can't be scratched. "The more I scratched it, the more it wanted to be scratched." This is the paradox of addiction.

Is processed food addiction another label for disordered eating?

Processed food addiction, in its various and overlapping forms, is such a subtle disease that it can lie dormant for quite some time. More importantly, I note with every processed food addict I treat, the disease manifests differently. For example, a patient may come in with symptoms of depression, anxiety, and stress because they have just lost their job, or they have moved from another country, or the person they want to be with has decided to be with someone else, or their pet has passed away. For most people, psychological, ethnic, financial, career, and social factors do influence how they are thinking or feeling, how much or how little they eat, or what actions they take. But for the processed food addict, these factors do not *drive* a person to start ingesting addictively. The addiction is purely physiological, and the person's body must in some way be able to physically ingest the considerable amount of processed food that is necessary to feed the addiction.

Hence, most people experiencing some turmoil in their life may increase their intake of processed foods because they are lonely or sad and because processed food alleviates some of their discomfort. However, unless the person has the physiological predisposition of addiction, they will be able to moderate and control their intake of processed foods, after a period of healing has occurred and their emotional turmoil has subsided. The point I am making here is that for those who are not real (severe) processed food addicts, the addiction does not progress. They can take it or leave it alone; they never experience the physical allergy and the mental obsession that comes with the disease of addiction. Saying this another way: for a non-PFA, it is the much saner choice to stop when they have had enough, but for the processed food addict, it is agony to stop once they get started.

Let's Share

It is Christmastime, and everyone is excited about the day. Family and friends are all around and have been enjoying the festivities and the food and drink that come with the day. Everyone is having a merry time, eating and drinking what they want as they catch up with each other.

However, Kelly is looking forward to her lunch. She has been on her diet (abstaining from sugar, flour, and wheat products) for a couple of weeks now. Lunch ends up being a bit later in the afternoon. As everyone sits down to eat, the thought crosses Kelly's mind: "It's 2:00 p.m. and I'm hungry. I've been good all day."

Kelly watches as everyone eats the turkey and roast veggies and gravy. She then, without a second thought, leans over and takes a portion of the baked vegetables and smothers it in gravy. Next she grabs a bread roll to soak up the gravy. She feels as though she has been rocketed into heaven. Finally, the anxiety and stress subside. She feels a part of the day at last.

Kelly continues eating as much as possible, even making excuses to go to the bathroom to vomit it up, or to wolf down the food she has hidden in a napkin.

Then the announcement comes from Dad: "I'm so full. Let's clean up and have dessert a bit later on."

Everyone agrees with him. Some may go and have a nap, others might play a board game, while others just sit and chat. They are completely satisfied with how much they have eaten.

But Kelly has only just started! She can't stop. She is beside herself, as she needs to keep eating.

The non-PFA never experiences the desire or need to continue ingesting processed food to alleviate the physical and emotional torment of *not* ingesting. For them, the more torturous decision is to keep on eating, but for the severe processed food addict, it is pure torture to stop. Processed food addiction in its various and overlapping forms takes on a chameleon-like role. One thing I do know: over time the disease of addiction progresses. It gets worse, never better.

Interestingly, the ambiguity of the term *food addiction* has been discussed with respect to substance abuse in numerous articles, using different terms when referring to processed food addiction as a substance use disorder.[2] Moreover, ambiguity has arisen in the diagnosis and treatment of addiction—in this case, PFA—regarding whether a medical-model approach or a social-model approach is better.

I believe in *and* implement an integrative approach, with effective results thus far.

---

[2] These articles have referred to addicts acquiring physical and psychological dependence on high fat, high sugar (HFHS) foods (Pivarunas, Conner, 2015); refined foods (Ifland, 2009); processed foods (Corsica & Pelchat, 2010; Moubarac, Parra, Cannon, & Monteiro, 2014; Raymond & Lovell, 2016; Stuckler, McKee, Ebrahim, & Basu, 2012); "highly processed foods" (Schulte, Avena, & Gearhardt, 2015); and "ultra-processed foods" (da Costa Louzada, 2015; Moodie, Stuckler, Monteiro, Sheron, Neal, Thamarangsi, 2013); and to "eating addiction" (Hebebrand et al., 2014) and "chocolate addiction" (Bruinsma & Taren, 1999).

Most importantly, the latest research on this topic highlights the need to be consistent universally in defining *processed food addiction* and *processed food addict*.[3] Explaining this will ensure consistency and clarity globally. Said in another way, as we come together and all use the same language, prevention and treatment methodologies will be constructively unified.

Perhaps I am a processed food addict, but I'm not as bad as the druggies and alkies, am I?

If I say I am a processed food addict, does it place me in the same class as a drug addict? All potential substance users, abusers, and addicts tend to downplay the severity of their addiction. Hence, as discussed previously, a potential processed food addict would prefer to be labeled something more temperate, such as *compulsive overeater, emotional eater, food abuser, anorexic, bulimic*—anything but *processed food addict*. It is also important to bear in mind that not everyone who is overweight is a processed food addict and that other forms of disordered eating do exist in society today. However, I work with patients who have tried most of the other remedies and yet still go back to ingesting more and more processed foods and find that now the malady has worsened.

Let's Share

I was working with a patient recently and this is how the conversation went.

> *I have a mixture of emotions in coming to terms with the disease concept. I don't like the word disease, so I think I'll use the word condition. I have a lot of fear and anxiety every time I think of it. My father is an untreated alcoholic and I never want to be like him or even associate in any way with him or with what he does.*

---

[3] Raymond, Kannis-Dymand & Lovell, 2017

I know it is not right for me to ingest processed foods, so I go for the healthier option. I make sure I use sweetener instead of sugar, order mocha zero-sugar treats or a smoothie, or buy a healthy version of a protein bar at my local organic vegan café. I just really want to be normal and not have this condition. Yes, my life is a bit unmanageable. I'm finding it harder to keep up my responsibilities at work—and on some days, I just don't make it.

But if I could just control my intake of processed foods and supplement with healthier options while losing weight, then I would be much happier, and able to cope with life.

We see that this persistent unwillingness to take responsibility for this malady hinders the processed food addict in seeking recovery. The individual tries to avoid facing up to having to build a new lifestyle that proactively treats the disease of processed food addiction. Thus, while in denial (and denial has a huge part to play in keeping the processed food addiction operational), the individual can continue to believe the illusion that "somehow, someday, some way, I'll be able to control and enjoy my processed food intake just like everyone else."

More often than not, PFAs are persuaded through marketing strategies, social media, advertising, and the like to believe that certain foods or beverages are "healthier option." Once again, the processed food addict is trying to control a substance they cannot control without sparking a craving for more. This opens up the door for denial by rationalizing "This is a much healthier option, at least I'm not eating fast food like such and such ..." Once more there is denial in this statement as they compare themselves to someone else to appear better, healthier or okay.

Taking this a step further, lurking in the addict's subconscious is the thought and feeling that "there will come a time and a day when I will be able to handle my processed food addiction *on my own.*" An addict can go to bed at night and wake up the next morning and think, "Gee, maybe I was making too big a deal out of all that addiction stuff.

I've been to thirty food anonymous meetings, abstained from sugar, flour, and wheat for three months, and lost 33 lb. (15 kg.), so perhaps I can control it now, or maybe I'm not one of those anymore?" This ability to avoid being re-addicted doesn't exist in the individual who is a severe processed food addict.

At an addiction medicine conference recently, I heard a simple statement: "The heart and soul of recovery from any addiction is an acceptance of the disease concept of addiction." Processed food addiction is not based on psychological distress, a dysfunctional upbringing, or a bad habit or compulsion. It is a bio-psycho-social-spiritual disease that incorporates all of one's life. Just like other substances of abuse, an addiction to processed food silently tears families apart, creates enormous economic burdens, and is a predecessor to other serious complications further down the path.

You may wonder why I repeat myself throughout my writing. The reason is, while I repeat myself, I live in an experienced belief that any reader who suffers from this malady may find some words of hope, eventually leading them toward seeking a solution to a malady they have no control over, whether ingesting processed foods or not. Hence, repetition is the mother of wisdom.

Chapter Three

A Paradigm of the Phases of Processed Food Addiction

> Holding your own
> against the disease of
> processed food addiction
> is like
> swimming in an ocean.
>
> The Author

Processed Food Addiction: An Analogy

In the early days of the disease, the addict will bob up and down, swimming joyfully, ingesting as much or as little processed food as they like. Then as time goes on, they start to get a bit tired, with not as much frolicking around in the water. Their weight starts to go on and stays on a bit longer, and it is more challenging to lose it.

Further along, the addict starts to be pulled under the water but is able to get back up on the surface again and starts to alternate between floating and dog-paddling—ingesting processed foods seems to become the norm now, even to the point of needing it to attend to some day-to-day activities.

Next, they get pulled under once again, and then again, and come up with a gasp to get some oxygen while just floating on top of the water. Processed food is now starting to dictate where they go, what they do, how they will do it, and what they will *not* do.

Yet further along, they go under and stay under for longer, coming up for a gasp of air, then going back under again. They fight to come back up with a huge gasp of air each time, thinking, "How do I get myself out of this mess?" Processed food starts to impact them mercilessly, tossing them around in many aspects of their daily lives. Their world is now one dichotomous time zone of black-and-white living: everything is about being good or being bad, happy or sad, euphoric or deeply depressed, hot or cold, yesterday or tomorrow.

This time they go under *and* stay under, and when they do bob up to the surface, they only breathe in small amounts of air, not enough to stay under for long but enough to keep on trying to find a way to get back up on top of the water, which they eventually do. The processed foods now control them. Each time they take some weight off, they put more back on; each time they find a new control method, it ends up failing. The time between binges is getting shorter and shorter, and the world becomes a dismal place if they have to keep on living like this—wishing for the end that just doesn't seem to come. Relentlessly, this merciless obsession with processed foods takes over, and they start to comprehend the fatal nature of their predicament.

In the end, the addict knows they are down for the count. They make one more attempt to get back up to the surface, and it's one more failure to stay above the water. No one really knows the reality of what's happening in the ocean. "Is this the end?" they may ask. "I can't get out of the ocean, but I can't stay here because I'm drowning."

The processed food addiction now masterminds the person's thinking, actions, and behaviors. They find they cannot live with ingesting processed foods, but they also know they cannot live without the processed foods. They are becoming desperate; people are starting to notice more and more as each day, week, month, and year rolls by. They have heard people talking about finally being able to lose weight and keep it off, even though it was becoming extremely hard to do so. Knowing this place very well, they just thought they could beat it where other people had failed. They thought they hadn't tried hard enough, or done enough, or known enough, vowing to try just one more time.

How many times have you said "just one more time"?

Some people float on the ocean, go under a couple of times, come up, and go under again over a very long period of time (decades, even). Others may do it for up to ten or twenty years. Still others hear about a solution and get hold of it—a buoy in the ocean—as soon as possible.

Where Are You in This Stormy Sea?

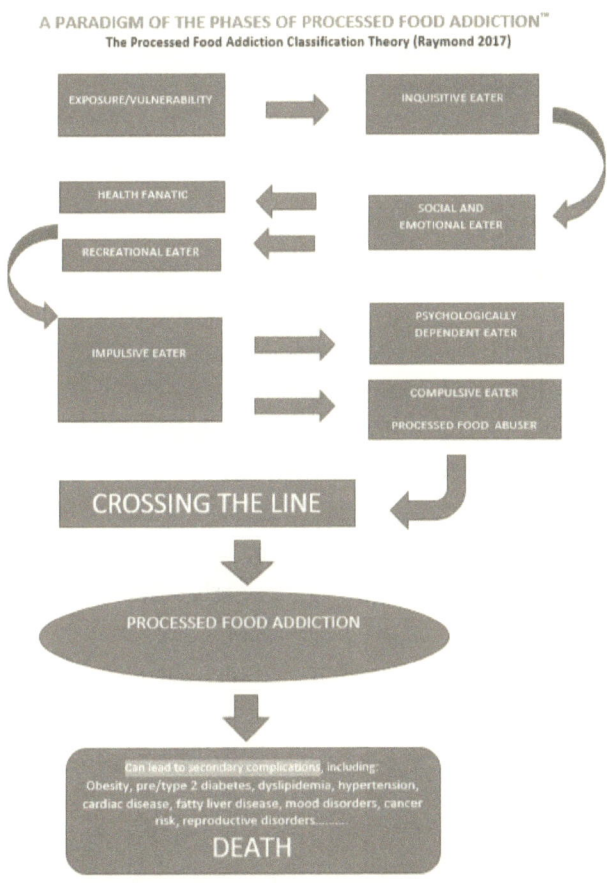

Exposure and/or Vulnerability to Addiction

Maureen Shares

> I loved being pregnant. I could eat what I wanted, when I wanted, where I wanted, and no one cared how thin or fat I was. I put on approximately 37 lb. (17 kg.) during my pregnancy. My go-to was a takeout joint that sold the best spiced hot fries, mashed potatoes, and gravy. I just couldn't get enough of it. That, and oh, also a cookie called a peanut butter dream bar. Fortunately for me, though, I knew I couldn't stomach this amount of stuff normally, so I thought I might as well enjoy this while I could.

Jill Shares

> I have started giving my two-year-old son Riley children's vitamins in the morning. I take vitamins, so I thought I would start him early. Luckily, they are easy to swallow and taste yummy, or so Riley says.

In today's society, it is hard to imagine there may be individuals under one or two years of age who have never ingested a processed, refined substance. It would be more believable to speculate that they have not *knowingly* ingested processed food, especially at such an early age (e.g., during fetal development). Literature has long postulated that mothers eat for two while pregnant, indulging in, for example, chocolate milkshakes or highly processed takeout food (excused by pregnancy cravings). Furthermore, if the mother eats a highly processed diet while breastfeeding, the early stages of a baby's life can also contribute to potential processed food abuse later in life. Likewise, sugars such as sucrose maltodextrin and corn syrup are added to baby formula. As the child grows through the toddler years, the local grocery shop has treatments for such things as teething or raised temperatures, each of which have hidden sugars in them, such as different flavored medicines and even sugar-laden vitamins that look like candies. However, there is still a lot of research to be undertaken to understand the effects of processed foods on the developing fetus and during the toddler years that goes well beyond the boundaries of this writing.

What most females do when pregnant, typically, is ingest more processed foods than they normally would. Hence, there would be no reason for a clinician to suggest that a pregnant mother should moderate or stop ingesting. Generally, at this stage, there is no difference between a non-processed food addict and a potential processed food addict. Just as it is for young Riley, a myriad of kid's vitamins are loaded with sugars. Will Riley grow up to be a processed food addict? Only time will tell.

The Inquisitive Eater

Joan Shares

> *Auntie Gladys always made the best shortbread cookies. She brought a large box of them whenever she came to visit.*
>
> *I loved visiting Aunt Gina when I was young, as she made the best spaghetti lasagna. The recipe was passed down from her grandmother.*
>
> *My friend at school brought in different treats that her mom made, and she offered them around to all of us. They were so sweet and so yummy.*
>
> *At birthday parties, there were always different types of food I had never tasted, so I tried to sample as many as I could, especially the ones that Olga said were special.*

Of course, most kids experiment and taste different foods; it is part of growing up. However, most birthday parties, christening parties, naming celebrations, and so on are enhanced with many processed food products to devour. At play here, to entice the youth of society into eating, are many factors, such as social, financial, ethnic, environmental, cultural, and traditional factors. And, of course, the smell and taste of processed foods. Last but most definitely not least, the marketing of such products has a huge influence on what a person ingests. Children in the twenty-first century are so much more exposed and quite vulnerable to ingesting copious amounts of processed foods. Only the other day I heard an advertisement on the radio about a teenager who had been stood up—her date did not show up, so what did she do? She shared how eating at a fried chicken franchise would help her get over it.

Then as children get older, education, discipline, moral teachings, and career prospects appear to also be jeopardized. Does this mean all the youngsters of today are potential processed food addicts? That's like saying everyone who was exposed to alcohol will become an alcoholic, which has not been the case thus far. Indeed, there is a lot of alcohol abuse, just as there is processed food abuse. But whether one will become a processed food addict remains unknown until much later on.

The Social and/or Emotional Eater

It is human to want to control and enjoy one's intake of processed foods. That is, to eat socially and not have to worry about the secondary consequences of gaining weight or facing health issues. I continually hear patients in clinic share that their parents, siblings, and friends eat processed foods all the time, "and they say they're social eaters." I hear "It's that time of the month and I just need some chocolate to calm me down." Usually, the next question is "Why can't I eat like my family and friends?"

Some patients attempt to define themselves as social eaters on the basis of how much or how little junk food they indulge in.

> *I usually have a dessert on Friday night with dinner.*
>
> *I make sure I limit the snacks I have when I go out.*

I might have a fast-food takeout on the weekend and then I quit.

More than a day of eating junk food is too much for me because it makes me feel zonked out, so I stop.

I only had such-and-such at the smorgasbord, and I felt so sick and queasy in my stomach and so full I had to stop.

Likewise, the emotional eater's statements are recognizable.

I feel so sad. I'm not as pretty or as thin as the other girls at school.

I can't play sports as well as them; I'm so clumsy and I feel bad.

My boyfriend and I had an argument, so I had to eat chocolate chip ice cream; it always makes me feel better.

And of course, there is social-media marketing, which enhances the connection between ingesting processed foods and feeling down. Once again, there is no reason to suggest the person cut down or stop ingesting processed foods. They may still not be a processed food addict at this stage, or they may be a potential processed food addict. Only time will tell.

The Controlling Eater-cum-Health Fanatic

Some people have never binged or ingested copious amounts of processed food. This may have come from certain moral, ethnic, or religious standards established in their homes, bringing about a certain discipline of controlling their consumption of processed food when they were growing up. Then we have another group of controlling eaters with different approaches toward their ingestion, such as excluding all sugars, or any foods that are white, or all flour and wheat products (especially the ones listed in the first three to six ingredients on the food label). Or eating only gluten-free products, or vegetarian, or Paleo, or raw foods, or the ketogenic diet ... The list goes on. These people may be able to control or moderate their processed food intake lifelong.

Eating-habit statements vary, such as,

> *Mom and Dad were vegans, so I just followed suit.*
>
> *Junk food was NEVER permitted in my home.*

Others say, "I don't like chocolate so I never eat it." Or "I saw the misery caused by Mom's excessive dieting and Dad's grossly overweight stomach. That motivates me to eat healthy all the time so I won't be like either of them."

> *My aunts all had diabetes (either type 1 or type 2), so I made sure I stayed away from all the junk food.*

Who is the processed food addict and who is the non-processed food addict? Only time will tell.

This is a good place to share about the *non*-bingeing eating cycles with processed foods, which is where people begin dieting. This starts them on a myriad of diets, for instance, a no-junk-food diet. These non-eating phases of the no-junk-food rule can take place at any time or at any point in the life of a non-PFA or a *potential* processed food addict. These phases may start at school (from ages six to twenty-six), in the sporting arena, at dance classes—wherever.

Quite often, I will hear a patient share details.

> *At school we all binged and then hid in the toilets so we could throw it up, but today all my friends are married, have kids, and don't seem to care about their weight. So, what is wrong with me? I am having trouble controlling my processed foods intake like my friends seem to be able to do, but I think I'm not trying hard enough, so with a little bit more effort and a new diet, I'm sure soon I will be just like them.*

Then there is the health fanatic, who uses excessive exercise to control their weight—notice I said *their weight*, not *their bingeing*. As we all know, a real processed food addict will not be able to control the amount of processed food they ingest, especially as the disease progresses, so they increase other control methods, in this case, exercise. Some people are fine with this; however, the potential processed food addict, over time, will end up ingesting way more than they can ever possibly burn off via exercise.

My patient Jo ingested junk food just like the other girls. However, she always seemed to want more when she stopped, so she started to exercise to control her weight. Then as Jo got older, she found she was always around 44 lb. (20 kg.) overweight, so she made up her mind to take up running. First, she just walked around her backyard. Then she increased her running time more than the distance she walked, until she could finally run 1 mile (1.6 km). Today, she runs six days a week and has done several half-marathons. Her goal and motivation are to one day do a whole marathon. She knows if she doesn't run, then she would be "as huge as an elephant," as she puts it.

Some people—those not addicted to processed food—can run or do any form of exercise until the end of time, but the potential processed food addict won't be able to keep this up long-term.

Some individuals use behavioral patterns to control their ingestion of processed foods. This could be a director of a large fashion empire or the CEO of a large investment company. They have what we call monthly processed food binge-benders. They can go a whole month without consuming processed foods, but at the end of the month, they have a four-day splurge from Friday to Monday. Then they taper off, go back to work until the end of the next month, and repeat the cycle.

Then we have another group of people who do not under any circumstances ingest processed foods from Monday to Friday, but then TGIF—"thank God it's Friday"—comes along and they go out with their colleagues for snacks, drinks, and a light dinner. Come Saturday and Sunday, they heavily ingest processed food, until late Sunday afternoon, when they know they have to taper off because they have work tomorrow. They may get away with this for months, years, or decades. But then they find that this pattern progresses from Monday to Thursday, finding it harder and harder to taper off; then it progresses from Monday to Wednesday, and so on.

Maryanne worked for a sporting goods company; she worked in merchandise two days a week and the other three days she did administration work. She loved her job. It kept her motivated during the week to stay off junk food, but come the weekend, it was a different story. She played in her company's Friday night volleyball team, which she loved. After the game, they always went out for late-night snacks and drinks. Then Saturday she refereed the local basketball competition and indulged in the barbecue and home-baked goodies. Come Sunday she could still eat what she wanted, as she had been good all weekend (volleyball and netball are very physical), so she rationalized that she didn't have to do anything to earn her binge—she deserved it. Come Monday, she got back on her diet until Friday again. This went on and on for Maryanne. As she got older, she tapered it down, had kids of her own, and found other things to live for. Whether or not Maryanne is a potential processed food addict remains to be seen down the track.

The Recreational Eater

I also see some phases of *recreational eating* happening around this time, that is, after people have yo-yoed back and forth between knowingly making healthy and unhealthy food choices. At this phase, processed food and the effects it provides are the center of attention. This person is all about chasing the effects that processed foods have to offer. They find that their lifestyle revolves around their eating activities just as much as going to work or to a sporting event or to the gym to burn off what they have indulged in. Uppermost in their mind is getting to this event and indulging in the effect. Their aim is to be like everyone else—ingesting as they see fit, as a normal part of life, and feeling great. Their motivation for living is always feeling great, being entertained (or being the entertainer), and enjoying life. They learn early on that overindulging in processed foods can numb all their problems and take the edge off life. They are the happy-go-lucky, roly-poly, or very cheerful person with a charismatic personality people want to be around. This overindulging can lead to short-lived amnesia, but when Monday comes around, the person who overindulged appears normal.

Most people don't think about processed food: where they can get it, how they will eat it (without anyone seeing them, of course), and how they can get rid of the evidence—not only the packaging but, the biggest symptom of all, the extra weight. They are just living until the next event, as one might say. They learn very quickly that this lifestyle makes you overweight but can also temporarily take away all your troubles, as you feel generally elated or content (even for a short time).

At this point, for some, worrying about their weight for the most part is a temporary concern. For others, putting on the weight is much worse than continually chasing a civilized processed-food orgy for which they begin to loathe the consequences. This may result in turning away from such events lifelong.

Bella's Case Study

I lived in Sydney and loved the nightlife, the lifestyle, and the never-ending invitations to be with my friends. Every Friday night, I would meet and support my colleague, who held cheesecake shop parties around the suburbs of Sydney. People who attended got to sample the different cakes and then pre-order one for an upcoming event.

I had been doing this for several months and always got to take home the leftovers. However, I noticed I was gaining quite a lot of weight. Over time, I started to urinate more at night, had a thirst that could not be quenched, and became more lethargic, to the point that attending work felt more and more impossible. I finally went to see my doctor and found out my blood sugar levels were very high; I walked out of the clinic with a type 2 diabetes diagnosis.

It seemed so surreal to me at first. I was in a blur as to how much my life was about to change: regular consults with an endocrinologist, attending diabetes support-group meetings, and basically changing my whole lifestyle.

Did Bella have a predisposition to diabetes? Did the Friday-night cheesecake parties put her over the limit? It doesn't really matter in the big scheme of things. One does not need to engage in processed-food parties to partake of processed foods in this way; it can take place anywhere that processed foods are available. Will Bella develop an aversion to junk food and treat and manage her diabetes effectively and consistently? Or might she be at a stage of denial, saying, "It isn't really that bad," and continuing on as before, trying to manage as best she can? Is processed food addiction underpinning Bella's type 2 diabetes symptomology while other complications continue to develop (such as hypertension and/or psychological distress)? Only time will tell.

Impulsive Eater

The personality trait of impulsivity is generally associated with all addiction-based diseases in one form or another and may be demonstrated to varying degrees in the majority of people who ingest processed foods. I am not here to analyze personality traits, as my expertise is primarily in the field of processed food addiction. At first, the impulsive eater may appear to be in the class of the social or emotional eater, but on impulse, she will begin to ingest processed foods for the effect. This may happen, for example, in any number of situations, including social celebrations, problems at home or at work, and financial upheaval. Most importantly, though, these impulsive binges tend to be controlled by a self-limiting condition. She may experience familiar signs and symptomology from the binge the night before, such as feeling wasted or having a *bingeover* (the aftereffects of ingesting so much processed food, similar to a hangover from a heavy night of alcohol). So she goes home to try to sleep off the ensuing backaches, headaches, nausea, and dry mouth. And of course, with the promise of "I'll never eat that again as long as I live" while she searches out the next diet ... to start on Monday.

Is she a processed food addict? Only time will tell.

Katrina's Case Study

Katrina knew she was a bit different from other people when it came to ingesting processed foods. She enjoyed them, especially when she was feeling a bit melancholy. However, Katrina could go on her latest diet and be "so good" for different lengths of time. But sometimes when she went out, she just couldn't help herself, especially at dessert time. She would not stop at one but usually went back three or more times and even got her boyfriend to pick her up an extra one.

She always felt horrible afterwards, but at the time, she just loved the feeling of sharing this part of the social occasion with other people. Not to mention it always made her feel a bit better—taking away the blues.

At times when she was at home, she would notice a package of creamy cookies in her cupboard. Katrina would open the package to have two with her afternoon cup of coffee, but just as she was about to gulp down the last two cookies, the phone would ring, and she would be called in to work. Katrina didn't eat the last two cookies, as her work was important to her, and knew she would eat them when she got home.

Katrina went to work, feeling okay. The cookies would have taken the edge off her mood, but she stopped ingesting them so she could go to work.

Next, potential processed food addicts start the period of eliminating processed foods, which may last until lunchtime, for a couple of days, for a few weeks or months, or even for the rest of their lives; but usually they are more likely to be what I term a *bender eater*. Now, this is an interesting character when it comes to a processed food addiction diagnosis. The bender eater follows a cyclical pattern of social and/or emotional eating, then of impulsive eating (bingeing), then of dieting (the no-junk-food rule) or abstinence (the elimination of processed foods), and then back to social and/or emotional eating.

This merry-go-round of behaviors and patterns of eating continues to go around and around throughout their life, painting a clear picture of ingesting, bingeing, and abstinence. This person may experience secondary complications, both physically and mentally, and they may die several years before their time. However, even though these people may find it challenging to change their eating behavior, they find they can do so with some form of help from a professional health clinician. Other assistance might be counseling to implement psychological methods such as mindfulness[4] and/or cognitive behavioral therapy (CBT) to moderate their overeating.[5] Alternatively, they might move interstate or overseas, meet the person of their dreams, or have another sufficiently strong reason to stop or moderate.

Rosie

Rosie loved processed foods and she loved life. However, she was a little bit chubby, not too much to write home about, but always a size or two bigger than her friends. Rosie always felt a bit *less than* and quite openly shared that she suffered from very low self-esteem. Rosie was always on a diet and could last several weeks at a time.

Then, passing the golden arches one day, she thought of an apple pie and a chocolate sundae, that was all. She quickly swerved into the parking lot, walked into the takeout, and ordered them, plus a burger and fries and a chocolate shake. She then sat and ate them in the car while watching all the other customers order their takeout for the

---
[4] Witkiewitz, Marlatt & Walker, 2005
[5] Beck & Beck, 2011

night ... but they kept driving. She knew she had eaten too much but vowed to go back on her diet on Monday, which she did, eliminating junk food once again.

Then, several weeks later, Rosie discovered her work hours had been cut back. She was not too happy about this, and on the way home she ducked into the 7-Eleven and picked up some takeout—two ice creams, a family-size chocolate bar, a hot meat pie with ketchup, chicken tenders, and an Italian sausage, which she devoured when she got home. Going to bed feeling horribly full, she decided she was going to seek some help to moderate her food intake and enroll in a self-esteem course she had seen advertised in the local paper. This, Rosie thought, would build her confidence while she looked for a full-time position.

Is Rosie a processed food addict? When can we say she has transitioned to actual physical dependency from the phases of psychological dependency or emotional dependency or compulsive eating? The fact is that this transition is completely individualized, as is the case with chronic illness; it is not exactly the same from one person to the next.

Processed food addiction manifests differently in each person being treated. Same disease, different manifestations. One individual may wake up one day and quit entirely with very little pain or secondary complications. Another may experience torturous withdrawal symptoms. Put another way, one individual can be psychologically dependent on processed foods, abusing processed foods time and again or rarely, but for whatever bio-psycho-social-spiritual reason may never progress to the physical-dependence phase.

If you are in doubt, stop ingesting processed foods for anywhere from 3 to 72 hours (if you can last that long). If you start to experience withdrawal symptoms, then there is a high probability you are physically dependent.

Angie

By the age of twenty-three, Angie had been admitted several times to a well-known eating-disorder clinic in Sydney. Several times, her body mass index (BMI) plummeted to the severe extremity of being underweight. In hospital, she managed to get some weight back on through transactional analysis and other behavioral and cognitive approaches. She was then admitted again (her fourth visit), got the weight back on, and approximately six months later found out she was pregnant. She never fought with food again; she had a baby daughter, married the father, and the rest is history. Angie may have had some symptoms of processed food addiction, but most importantly, she was able to seek the medical help that supported her change with positive future outcomes.

These patterns illustrate two major offshoots of disordered eating: psychological dependence and physical dependence. The person has learned to seek the effects to deal with their psychological distress (depression, anxiety, or stress), or they engage in short feasts, consuming large amounts of calories. The second may be labeled a compulsive eater (also sometimes called a binge eater). Purging is not always the aftermath and becomes less and less viable as an option as the consequences progress and are more detrimental; hence, secondary complications—including obesity, diabetes, heart disease, and fatty liver syndrome—start to play an important part as an appendage to the primary cause, the processed food addiction.

The role impulsivity plays in the disease of addiction is still being debated. What I have experienced in the clinic with the majority of patients is that as we treat the malady of addiction (by eliminating the cause—processed foods), the consequences dissipate substantially over time. If only the consequences (e.g., weight, depression, anxiety, type 2 diabetes (t2d), hypertension, and more) are treated, then the cause is still operational and will present again, sooner or later.

Psychological Dependence

The euphoric effect is what's most important when a person comes to depend on processed foods psychologically, and even more so when they do so physically. The motivation of these individuals is pain—chronic pain such as back pain (e.g., what's been prescribed doesn't even take the edge off), emotional pain (e.g., feeling depressed because they can't find anyone to love them), or anxiety (e.g., their work is becoming bigger than they can handle). I am sure you can think of many similar situations happening in your life at this minute.

With both psychological and physical pain, the individual will ingest processed foods (graze on them throughout the day or binge) to cope with the stresses, aches, and pains of life. The situation is thus a means to relieve physical, emotional, and mental suffering.

At this stage, over-the-counter medications can come in to help ease the pain (self-medication). Some people will vary their self-medication regime, while others come to understand that ingesting processed foods gives them the same effect of what I call *emotional anesthesia*. For the processed food addict, the latter becomes the preferred choice of relief, as clearly it takes a lot less time to get processed food than to go to a drugstore (pharmacy), with the added bonus of not having to see the middleman (the doctor)—*and* it can be done in secret.

However, self-medication may also be a potential warning, the bridge needed for multi-comorbidity, bringing about more problems. The potential processed food addict's mental problems, ranging from general anxiety disorder to depression or depressive disorders (and a myriad of mental diagnoses in between), may start off acutely, becoming more chronic as the addiction progresses. Here, processed foods can serve as a temporary fix by quieting the brain down. Of course, this can lead to dependency later on.

As time goes on, this becomes the norm for a potential processed food addict—chasing the effects produced by processed foods to relieve the pain, any pain: physical pain, mental pain, life pain. Believe it or not, this is their only known reality. Even though they understand the consequences of each binge, they cannot discern fantasyland from reality. Their processed food addiction lifestyle is their reality. Once again, the restlessness, irritability, and discontentment set in, and the only relief they know (like in the movie *Groundhog Day*) is to ingest processed foods, again, which they see others all around them doing with impunity.

The extremes of this stage range from the individual who has to stop off at the local 7-Eleven each day to ingest processed foods in order to function—meaning, face whatever awaits her at home. This might be that her husband is running late so she has to pick up the kids when she has something else planned, one of the children has fallen off his bike and broken his arm (medical expenses, emotions and fears to soothe, and a waste of time), or the dishwasher has broken and can't be fixed. Loss of time especially adds fear, as it will take away from the eating time she had planned.

It doesn't take much to envision the obesogenic environment that abounds in lower-socio-economic areas, where people rely on cheap feasts to help anesthetize the reality of their situations.

And similarly, we can imagine the well-to-do areas, where people portray what we call "functional processed food addicts getting by." They appear to have it all together, but for some, the appearance on the outside changes from one month to the next: the weight goes up and the weight goes down! They may spend all their money attending health retreats and day spas, which promote a controlled environment to "get back on track" through strict dieting, detoxification, and body cleansing methods, because they can afford it. Plus they have the affluence to not be judged, with lots of people around to enable them. But for how much longer? As long as society says it is okay to be overweight, we will adjust our clothing sizes and the models in the windows (which is already happening) so we look like the norms these days. This gives society the permission to say, "It is okay to overindulge in processed foods; everyone else is."

For a proportion of people, a daily numbing using processed foods is needed to deal with their daily way of life, whether in planned bingeing, grazing throughout the day, or nocturnal ingesting. Do these people go on to become *severe* processed food addicts? Only time will tell.

A Case Study

Growing up, Sharon always felt empty inside. Even though she had an okay upbringing, there was still an emptiness, "a hole in the soul," which she had felt as long as she could remember. Dad was quite obese, while Mom tried to cope with the situation as best she could. Brother was physically present but didn't interact much. Sharon, who was also overweight as a child, knew she was different as soon as the kids at school called her chubby.

When she went to university, she lost quite a lot of weight and boys started to take a bit more notice of her. Sharon liked this, thinking it was the answer, so she got in and out of dysfunctional relationships, trying to keep herself on the diet merry-go-round, with relationships also producing the effect she'd sought through processed foods.

After a time, Sharon's anxiety increased and self-medication began. Not long after, prescription meds followed to take care of the psychological distress (depression, anxiety, and stress) that seemed to plague her more and more each day. She could not get off this roundabout of dieting, bingeing, boyfriends, and pills. Alcohol also played its part: she began drinking to anaesthetize the pain. The effects of the alcohol seemed to last longer than ingesting the processed food. However, she always made her way back to her preferred elixir—processed foods.

As she continued to seek toxic relationships, she knew subliminally that her default solution of processed foods and alcohol would fix it. Stress at university? Then pills *and* processed foods would fix it. Loneliness set in: even though she caught up with friends often and played beach volleyball once a week, she was still lonely. But processed foods and a movie binge would fix it. "No one can see me now in the darkness of the cinema."

Any excuse to ingest the processed foods was good enough. This became Sharon's reality. Weight went up and weight went down (sometimes a little, sometimes a lot), only for her to gain more the next time around, with more and more excuses to keep the addiction alive *and* progressing.

Jess

Jess lived in a well-to-do city area. Tall and at a normal weight, she appeared on the outside to live an ideal lifestyle. Her husband was a very well-to-do CEO of an electrical company. The children were in their late teens, attending private schools and a prestigious university. Their house was immaculate. However, Jess had a secret. When her husband left for work, Jess would start eating: a packet of cookies in the pantry, then to the fridge, finishing off last night's pavlova, then heating up some leftover lasagna. As the effect of the processed foods kicked in and the flavors and aromas rose to her head, Jess felt good.

All the things that she had to do for the rest of the day were now achievable. She even wondered whether she had been making too big a deal of it, but first she just had to slip to the bathroom. Five minutes, it was done. No weight gain. More importantly, no one knew.

This lifestyle continued for a few more years. However, it became increasingly hard for Jess to stop at the amount of food she used to eat. The amount of processed foods required to get that effect—that feeling of sedation—kept on increasing. Sleeping pills didn't seem to be working like they used to; her antidepressant meds didn't seem strong enough.

As the days went on, she felt even worse; waking up to face another day like this was torture. Now her binges were lasting much longer. It took more time to get the extra food and to justify to her husband where all the money was going. The binges and purges increased to up to four times a day, leaving Jess feeling more and more exhausted. Keeping up this double life took its toll. Jess's husband started pressuring her to go back to work and pestering her as to why she was not as much fun anymore. "Why do you take everything so damn seriously?" For a moment, Jess thought that going back to work would give her a reason to stop doing what she was doing.

Perhaps it will; perhaps it won't if she is a *real* processed food addict.

Emily

Then there was Emily, who lived in in a smaller town in northern New South Wales, just a twenty-minute drive from larger suburbia. She was a well-respected church member and an avid member of the community, cooking for all the church functions and organizing charity days. She had a loving husband who would do anything for her. However, Emily was extremely overweight. This was easily justified, as she was loved by her community, who knew they could always rely on her to do the catering. Emily was diagnosed with t2d in her thirties. Her mother had been a type 1 diabetic for as long as Emily could remember.

Emily tried many diets and ways to lose the extra weight. She knew it wasn't healthy to stay at her weight, and her diabetes caregiver was always calling her on it. "You need to lose the weight, Emily, or your diabetes will progress and other secondary complications will follow."

But in a small country town, no one judged her for her weight. In fact, she was known for her baking and everyone loved her for all the food she made and baked. She thought to herself, "I don't need to change at all. I have done all right thus far. I'll be fine. I'm sure of it. Plus, the church and community can't function without my help."

As time went on, Emily had to have hip surgery and then, twelve months later, another hip replacement. Then she was put on medication for her t2d, with more complications following: hypertension, gall bladder removal, and fatty liver disease.

When Emily reached her late fifties, feeling more breathless each day, she was still baking and ingesting processed food like it was going out of style. Is Emily a "real" processed food addict?

As time went on, Emily decided she didn't want to live that way anymore. She sought help through her local diet club and had help from a clinician to change her thoughts and behaviors. For example, she hung a huge sign on the pantry door that read "NO, Emily, it's not worth it."

Now she has changed her daily routine so as not to pass the bakeries, and she only does the food shopping once a week, with a list. She takes daily medications for her blood pressure and her t2d is mostly under control. She walks most days, which has helped her breathing enormously.

Emily's community has only encouraged her to keep going with "whatever you are doing." She may not do all the baking (and tasting) now, but instead she plays the church organ and helps out in the community shop selling handmade crafts. Every now and again, she does a bit of baking, but she also has someone to help her stop after the taste test and not be the one and only taste-tester.

Is Emily a real processed food addict? Indeed, she has quite a few of the symptoms of processed food addiction, but not enough to impair her life. Thus, she was able to do something about it. Whether Emily crosses the physiological line or not, only time will tell.

Some people do cross the line into addiction, while the majority of people do not; they can still "get away with it" for now. Of late, though, I am seeing that more often than not the majority of potential processed food addicts have to try to temper their consumption of processed foods or they too could be in the progressive stages of processed food addiction.

Moreover, Emily had not experienced that torment of the mind that appears in the devilish processed food addict personality. I see this can sometimes be the point where a person is pushed over the line to physiological and psychological manifestations of addiction. As my patients call it,

> *that voice that never shuts up, the one that gets louder and louder, drives me crazy with innuendos of how I'm such a failure and how hopeless and unworthy I am. Sometimes I think I'm going crazy, but when I ingest some processed food, it quiets down for a bit, only the time it shuts up after a binge is getting shorter and shorter.*

This voice I believe plays a huge role in keeping the processed food addict in denial.

Compulsive Eater

Non-PFAs (the ones who can make up their mind to stop once they've had enough) cannot for the life of them understand when a person says, "I can't stop ingesting processed foods." Of course, society accepts the addictive nature of alcohol, cocaine, heroin, amphetamines, and so on. However, it seems to blame the substance, not the addict. But processed food addiction is seen as different because everyone everywhere ingests processed foods and only a low percentage are real processed food addicts. Even so, I tend to be a bit more skeptical these days, with the way the obesity epidemic is sweeping the world—not to forget the increase in other chronic diseases related to obesity, including diabetes, hypertension, and cardiovascular disease.

Paramount to any addiction is the tendency to downplay its degree of severity. Hence, it is much easier and more acceptable in society to be a compulsive eater than to be a processed food addict.

Using the term *compulsive* can be seen as an attempt to find an easier, softer way to deny the truth that one might be a processed food addict, which would mean a whole lot of change, undertaking a new lifestyle. Hence, this allows the potential processed food addict to stay in denial (there's that word again)—living in fantasyland, the illusion, delusion, and obsession that somehow, someday, some way they will be able to ingest and enjoy their processed foods like everyone else. Here is where the problem lies.

It is a common misperception that addiction is a choice—a psychological, behavioral, or moral problem—and all you have to do is stop, or at least take measures to learn how to stop. It is far easier to accept being a compulsive eater, an emotional eater, a recreational eater, or even a psychological eater, or being diagnosed with "a binge eating disorder" than to face having a chronic disease known as *addiction*.

It has often been said that a compulsive person can moderate their habit, but an addict can only eliminate.

Researchers still debate the nature and/or nurture underpinnings of addiction; even the definition of addiction is controversial.

Processed food addiction is not simply the result of a compulsion, a psychological tendency, the manifestation of parental neglect, or any other reason one can conjure up, but is a whole way of life. So much more can be written about this topic; however, it is beyond the scope of this book for now.

Already I have observed from the literature that once some people start ingesting processed foods, they can't stop, or as the expression goes in recovery from processed food addiction circles, "they lose control."

Exciting research in the fields of genetics and addiction is looking at the neuronal pathways and the chemistry of the brain and how they work in relation to addiction. This may provide us with a much clearer picture for prevention and treatment methods in the future. I still wholeheartedly believe that addiction has a large genetic component. Hypothetically, one day we will isolate just a small snippet, a polymorphism of a gene, and be able to test potential candidates for addiction (in this case, processed food addiction), and of course implement strategies for prevention rather than treatment. My ultimate dream would be to get all the professionals in the world to spend time investigating this genotype, as it will take a lot of economic power to accomplish this. For now, I will keep it simple and not get too caught up in the methodology but concentrate more on the results (that is, what's working).

Case Study

Jenny has always had trouble with her food intake. Ever since she can remember, she was a little bit on the chubbier side and always found it easy to put on weight. She did a few diets growing up, listening to the never-ending heartbreaking comments of people she met: "You have such a pretty face. If only you could lose a couple of pounds."

So, with all the willpower she could muster, it was one more diet, followed by one more binge.

Then she heard about compulsive overeating. She went to a few support-group meetings and really identified: these people also found it hard to control how much they ate. Together they helped each other to eat only three moderate meals each day. It seemed pretty simple, and the term *compulsive overeater* explained to Jenny what was wrong with her.

Jenny continued to attend these support fellowships, got abstinent from compulsive overeating, and felt better, as at least people could understand her and she was no longer alone. But she could not stop compulsive overeating long-term.

Jenny tried to change her environment. She was a nurse at the local public hospital doing a lot of shift work. Sometimes she would get bored, especially in the early hours of the morning. All the patients were sleeping and there was limited staff on the night shift. Jenny often felt anxious, stressed, and tired. Having a couple of bars of chocolate always pepped her up. Some nights, when the anxiety and craving got pretty bad, she would sneak in and take advantage of the medications available for the patients on her ward. It gave her extra relief, she said, and she thought she wasn't hurting anyone and that it was more important for her to show that she was coping with work. Plus, it helped to fill in the anxiety between meals, as she was now eating three moderate meals per day as her newfound friends did.

Physiological changes may or may not have occurred in the compulsive overeater or the psychologically dependent eater as I have defined them above. The two symptoms I look for in an addiction diagnosis are tolerance and withdrawal, which I have previously discussed under "What does a sick brain mean in the context of processed food addiction?" If a person needs to increase the amount of processed foods she ingests to get the hit—the desired effect—then her tolerance level has increased, which may or may not be accompanied by withdrawal symptoms (depression, anxiety, stress, headaches, backaches, anger, fear, doubt, and panic attacks).

If someone is addicted to a certain substance, she generally develops a tolerance to that substance. However, she may not become automatically physically dependent on the substance (in this case, processed foods). The paradigm of processed food addiction holds that both compulsive overeaters and persons who are psychologically dependent on processed foods are *abusers*. That is, they both abuse processed foods.

In today's society, whether or not a person will cross the somewhat invisible line to addiction—that is, become physiologically dependent on processed foods—cannot be predicted; and it is also beyond the scope of this writing. A processed food addict will know they have crossed the invisible line to physiological dependence only when it has happened. What keeps the disease progressing is, once again, denial (there's that word again): hoping against hope they will be able to control and enjoy their processed food intake like everyone else.

Unfortunately, the person is abetted by the ignorance of our world today, which does not comprehend the difference between sane eating and processed food *addiction*. Information such as that contained in these pages will, I believe, bring about earlier diagnoses. I look forward to sharing, in the near future, what to do when it looks as though one is staring down the cookie jar of a processed food addiction diagnosis.

Crossing the Invisible Line into Addiction

How does one cross the line from psychological dependency or compulsive eating to a condition of being physically dependent on processed foods? Each person is unique, and from what I continue to clinically observe, some individuals start to bottom out (lose all control of their intake of processed foods) in their early thirties to forties, while others run the gauntlet when they are over the fifty-year mark.

However, I predict this is all about to change, as I see a huge global revolution taking place, especially in our youth of today. The majority of children these days in first- and even second-world countries are raised on highly refined and processed foods. Does this mean processed food addiction will present itself much earlier, or does it mean there will be a lot more of this malady globally? When treating processed food addiction, I am forever mindful of such an enormous change happening before our very eyes. Prevention is the best line of treatment, and hopefully as we all become more informed about this disease, more can be done to prevent it.

As a side note, the war on processed foods appears to be playing out quite bizarrely in a very similar fashion to what we experienced in the war on tobacco (Brownell & Warner, 2009).

In the twenty-first century, there appear to be more and more potential processed food addicts showing signs and demonstrating symptoms of addiction in their mid-twenties and early thirties. What is most important to acknowledge at this stage is that once the line has been crossed to physical dependency, the processed food addict will experience all the facets that go with withdrawal—the physical and mental anguish that follow when processed foods are eliminated from a person's system.

Interestingly, one type of ingester is emotionally addicted to processed foods and can seem to sometimes abuse them and at other times not. But for some reason, this person never becomes physically dependent. So, the question I would ask is "How does someone know if they have an inherent physical allergy to something that makes them dependent on processed foods, and a mental obsession that condemns them to go on eating?"

One of the simplest tests is to try to stop ingesting processed foods. After a period of time (say one to five days after your last bite), assess whether you experience a sequence of physical and mental signs and symptoms. You may have to try this once or twice. If you do experience such symptoms, then I would undoubtedly say you are clearly on the road (if you are honest with yourself) and you may have already crossed the line into a dependence on processed foods. Some people may be able to stop for a week, a month, six months, or even a year or more. However, once this line of physical dependence is crossed, then, yes, I would suggest strongly that untreated processed food addiction is at hand. If it is left untreated, medical complications abound, progressing to a fatal diagnosis, which is typical of many chronic diseases.

Thus, once again, it is pertinent to remember and reiterate that our reactions to processed foods are highly individualized and there should be more latitude in regard to the tremendous variation among processed food addicts.

I hope the sharing of personal experiences and case studies thus far has echoed this variation. Clinicians implementing valid and reliable methods, such as the DSM-5 Other or Unknown Substance Use Disorder Criteria, to discern the symptom count and apply a severity level indicator (mild, moderate, or severe) is most definitely a step in the right direction.[6]

The Yale Food Addiction Scale has also been shown to be a valid test battery.[7] What is most encouraging to me as a professional in this field is that this book may be a keystone in bringing about more awareness of and understanding that processed food addiction is a unitary disease of addiction.

Another trend I see happening with new patients is an increase in the number who have attended 12 step fellowships and yet still relapse time and time again. I think inadvertently there is a message suggesting that doing the 12 steps will stop them from ingesting, drinking, or using. They seem to think they are cured, or if they attend the fellowships they will have an immunity to processed foods. Even though the literature of AA states that they will never be cured, what I do know is that in the heart of hearts of *all* addicts there is this fallacy that somehow, someday, they will turn around and ingest processed foods like a lady—and finally appear to be normal, that is, control and enjoy processed foods just like everyone else.

---

[6] American Psychiatric Association, 2013
[7] Gearhardt, Corbin & Brownell, 2016

In the early days of AA, in their desperation, potential alcoholics came to understand that there was something more going on than just stopping drinking. They all learned they had a chronic illness and that the only way to get well and to stay well was to treat it daily. Primarily, at first, eliminating the substance, receiving the medical treatment as required, and then learning how to live a spiritual way of life by practicing the 12 steps in their entirety.

Quite often, I hear a person say, "K-L, just take me through the *Big Book* of AA and that will fix me," or "Help me control ingesting processed foods." Furthermore, individuals working in professional roles acknowledge they have high symptomology of processed food addiction and often say, "Teach me how to treat myself." That's like someone with a chronic disease, for example, t2d or heart disease, in the early stages saying, "Teach me about my heart" or "my diabetes" and then walking away with the information and trying to fix themselves.

This disease of PFA is cunning, baffling, and powerful, and its goal is a fatal prognosis. So it will do anything to keep the addict in denial, that is, look for an easier, softer way to try to manage their symptoms on their own. "Yes, I'll put the processed foods down all right, but I'm not changing anything else. My intelligence, self-knowledge, and self-reliance will keep me going and on track to control and moderate my ingestion of processed foods."

It may work for a while, but long-term and permanent abstinence with peace of mind is a far way off if the potential addict still subliminally believes they are enough or searches for other psychodynamic or scientific theories to one day cure themselves.

CHAPTER FOUR

A Non-PFA Versus a PFA

The Case of Joy, a Non-PFA

Joy lost a loved one and started to ingest more and more processed foods, finding emotional comfort in them while she experienced the grieving process. For Joy, ingesting processed foods took away some of the pain she associated with grief, including depression, anger, sadness, loneliness, isolation, worry, and fear. However, as Joy's grieving healed, down the road she was able to cut down her intake of processed foods to a more socially acceptable level. Joy did *not* progress to the addiction stage, as she does not have the physiological makeup of addiction. The difference is that phenomenon of craving that compels a processed food addict to ingest more and more often to relieve the physical and mental agony of not ingesting processed foods.

Thus, for the social and/or emotional eater, not ingesting more and more processed foods actually makes her feel better than continuing on, which for Joy is common sense—it's rational thinking.

Now what about a person who is predisposed to processed food addiction? They too go through the grieving process when they lose a loved one and may ingest some processed foods to help them heal from the pain of the grieving process. However, as time passes, their desire and craving to ingest processed foods becomes more powerful, and they are unable to stop because of the agonizing withdrawal symptoms and an even stronger desire to still ingest them. For this person, it is a much more agonizing choice to *not* ingest the processed foods—that is, to *stop*—than to keep going.

The Case of Caryn, a Severe Processed Food Addict

I was full of fear and loneliness at the loss of my lifelong partner. I literally sobbed on the bed, weeping as the fear and hopelessness enveloped me. How was I going to survive without him? I tried to cut down my processed foods intake, as I knew they were affecting my moods and not helping; however, I felt hopeless. So, then I gave myself permission to eat them, as I was so heartbroken.

My weight started to go up and I knew I had to stop. For some reason, I was wanting more and more of them. Knowing I was going down to the bakery to get some things for my breakfast always helped me to get out of bed. But then I found myself buying so much more extra processed foods—my favorite being long cream donuts, sausage rolls I could reheat, and to save some money, I would buy cakes that were made fresh and on sale for birthdays. This helped me through the day. I always felt better when I was eating them, but I knew I had to stop.

Even before Frank passed on, I had tried many things to lose weight and stop ingesting these foods that kept calling to me. Frank even helped me on my diets, but I knew I had been hopeless before, nothing worked long-term, and now it was quite evident that nothing had changed.

Seeking help from my doctor, I told him about my sadness and anxiety and my overindulgence. He gave me a script for some antidepressants. That didn't even help.

Over the ensuing nine months, my weight skyrocketed. I felt I had lost myself and thought I was going crazy.

I then went to see a psychiatrist, who quietly informed me I was putting too much pressure on myself while I was grieving. He suggested I was giving my inability to stop overindulging at this time too much importance in the big scheme of things of losing Frank. He said, "Just treat it as a fundamental social grace at this time in your life. Go out with your church folk and enjoy some home-baked goodies. Just have two like your friends and stop. You will feel better and, more importantly, you won't be alone. Here is a script for some sleeping tablets. You may take one with a light snack before you go to bed, aiding you to sleep better."

I paid $217 for this consult, which only added salt to my wounds.

So, I then went and saw the priest who led the funeral service at the time of Frank's passing. After I told him what was happening, he wrote on a piece of paper, "I promise I will not overeat on junk food ever again." He got me to sign it and write it out ten times before I ate breakfast, ten times before I ate lunch, and ten times before I ate dinner.

To me, when I looked at what I was writing, I only saw meaningless words. I did not have any willpower to stop, so I opened the freezer and finished off the tub of chocolate chip ice cream I had bought that morning. I felt hopeless.

In their own specialist fields, my doctor, psychiatrist, and priest were very accomplished.

However, in understanding the disease of processed food addiction, I started to identify with others who also suffered from my condition (which was what I first called it). When it came to helping me stop, or even cut down, my ingesting of processed foods—a substance that I undoubtedly could see was affecting me physically and mentally and destroying my soul, they were just as powerless as me. I fought this disease for several more years, well after my dear loved one had passed.

It is not unusual for a more mature individual to come through my doors. My youngest patients are in their twenties and my oldest patient turned eighty-three while recovering from this disease, which is similar to alcoholism: age is not a primary predictor of whether one is a processed food addict or not. Unfortunately, these individuals have gone on to suffer for way longer than was needed.

As one patient shared, "The word I used to describe my disease when it was active (before I found recovery) was *relentless*, for the mental anguish of whether I was ingesting processed food or not never seemed to end!"

The disease concept of alcoholism and drug addiction primarily emerged early in the nineteenth century. However, it wasn't until 1956 that the American Medical Association (AMA) declared alcoholism to be an illness.[8] This was several decades after the late W. D. Silkworth, MD, posited the disease theory of alcoholism, accompanied by the aphorism "The alcoholic suffers from an allergy."[9] Blessedly, I hope recovery will be available today in one's much earlier years, as I continue to have an optimistic mentality. It will not take this long for the disease of processed food addiction to be acknowledged as a chronic illness.

Furthermore, the AMA, accompanied by other medical systems and organizations, formally called addiction a disease in 1987, and in 1997, over four decades after first calling alcoholism an illness, the AMA further endorsed the dual classification of alcoholism by the International Classification of Diseases under both psychiatric and medical headings.[10]

I think I know my problem, but my solutions are not working. Why are my solutions not working?

There are a lot of dangers in searching for a solution without really understanding the disease of processed food addiction. I understand

---

[8] Leshner, 1997
[9] *Alcoholics Anonymous*, 1939
[10] Leshner, 1997

that while you have been reading these pages and digesting the phases of processed food addiction, you have been looking for answers for yourself. "An addiction to sugar, high fat, salt, wheat, flour, chocolate, food and so on ... and how to overcome it" is often discussed on billboards, in movies, on TV, in social media, and in magazines of all descriptions. The list goes on, with the latest diet, weight-loss group, healthy meals delivered to your door, gym memberships, self-help books, and cooking tips. In fact, the latest weight-loss gimmick at the time of this writing in Australia is a lollipop that guarantees a decrease in hunger, with the ultimate goal being—wait for it—weight loss. It was accompanied by a picture of the most in-the-news celebrity sucking on it.

Well, that's just the point I am making. If one is a real processed food addict, there is no quick fix. There is no *one* answer, as the disease of processed food addiction is cunning, baffling, and powerful, manifesting differently from one person to the next. Yes, same disease, same substance, but different ways the potential processed food addict has tried infinitely to prove that somehow, someday, they can control and enjoy their eating of processed foods just like everyone else.

What I continue to find in treating processed food addicts is that they already know (or so they are quite quick to inform me) that they are compulsive overeaters, bulimics, emotional eaters, and the like. They know their problem is that they just haven't found the right answer yet to fix themselves. And their problem is with "this God thing" in the 12 step fellowships, or not getting some spiritual angle that everyone seems to talk about, or, or, or!

Unfortunately, many real processed food addicts only make the first surrender—that is, they give up individual rigidities. For example, they might allow themselves to go where processed food is served or go out with family and friends more often. Once surrender takes place, they feel at ease and admit to being defeated by ingesting processed foods. This is underpinned by a degree of hopelessness and despair, leading to an attainment of surrender, admitting they haven't been able to beat it, resulting in the reduction of their ego and finally conceding the need for outside help.

However, this act of surrender comes with many problems. In reality, it may be more like *submission*, where the individual only accepts reality at a conscious level, which differs from *surrender*, where the individual accepts the truth at the subconscious level. If an individual stays in the submission stage, the fight is still going on. On the outside, they may seem to be beaten, but internally they are still in denial. Presently, they may be empty of processed foods, telling whoever will listen, "I feel better, think better, work better. Don't know why I didn't do this sooner."

Having been in this game for a while now, I give a wry smile, as I have seen this too many times before. I know this person is like a little girl whistling in the dark to stay hopeful, fooling themselves. Internally, they would give anything to go out to a buffet and eat all they wanted and get away with it. Surrender at the conscious level (submission) is about the person only just resigning themselves to the fact that they are a processed food addict, with the inner turmoil ever present. Sometimes, I call it sitting on the fence. One leg on one side of the fence is swaying toward "Yes, I am a processed food addict," while the other leg is dangling on the other side of the fence, saying, "I don't want to be a processed food addict—ever." When a person accepts at the subconscious level the reality that they have a chronic condition, with an inner knowing that they will never be able to ingest processed foods, then the residual fight is over.

This leads to an understanding that the disease is lifelong and that there will be a need for outside help for an indefinite period of time. Unfortunately, many individuals who tend to sit in between the moderate to severe symptomology of processed food addiction only make the first surrender and inevitably do not experience all the freedom, joy, and serenity that come when their disease goes into remission. Because of this inward fight still happening—that is, not surrendering to the truth (it is nice to say something about the opposite of denial)—they are often miserable and/or go back to ingesting processed foods sooner or later. Knowing the importance of discerning whether a potential processed food addict is either submitting or surrendering is vital in addiction diagnosis and treatment. Hence, I have further simplified the subject matter of submission versus surrender in chapter 3.

Of course, relapse is understandable in all chronic diseases, and processed food addiction is no different. However, when the patient is already in treatment and has been living a way of life that promotes recovery for some time, this new norm tends to ultimately dominate, leaving times of relapse fewer and further in between. The ultimate goal in my practice is what I call "longevity of recovery," which equates to abstinence with peace of mind being the norm for a processed food addict.

I have covered but a bare beginning in this writing for now, and I look forward to sharing more in depth regarding this subject matter at another time. Meanwhile, I encourage you to look for the similarities and not the differences. What can you identify with? *"Is this me?"* And not so much "I'm different because ... "

Hopefully, I have provided you with a lot of food for thought thus far.

Chapter Five

Grief and Recovery

When I stop ingesting processed foods, I always feel a lot of grief and sadness. It feels kind of like what I read about withdrawal from other things like alcohol or nicotine.

Why?

Grieving also plays an enormous part in recovering from a chronic disease.

The Five Stages of Grief

The five stages of grief are denial, anger, bargaining, depression, and acceptance.

Denial

The first stage of grieving helps us to survive the loss of not being able to eat like the majority of people, one day at a time. To see people eating whatever they want, whenever they want, wherever they want feels like rubbing salt onto a wound. When you feel you are being judged or persecuted for something that is not even your fault, you feel bad, sad, frustrated, and angry. In this stage, the world of socialization can become meaningless and overwhelming. Life makes no sense—it's like, "What's the use?"—especially in a changing society that promotes takeout foods as the norm.

Takeout food is economical, legal, and readily obtainable in a world where people appear to find it easy to control while enjoying their ingestion of processed foods. The processed food addict can be in a state of shock and denial. We can go numb and wonder how we can go on, if we can even go on. Why should we go on if nobody has to do this like we do? No one really understands. At first, we try to find a way to simply get through each day. Denial and shock help us to cope and make survival possible. Denial helps us to pace our feelings of sadness and grief of detoxing from processed foods.

> *There is a grace in denial. It is nature's way of letting in only as much as we can handle.*
>
> *(Elisabeth Kübler-Ross)*

As you accept the reality of being a processed food addict and start to seek answers, you are unknowingly beginning the healing process. You are actually facing reality for the first time without a substance to lean on, and the denial is beginning to fade. However, as you proceed, all the feelings that were denied begin to surface. If one were to sit down and process the work Christmas party, one would see all the different feelings, thoughts, and behaviors arising that are usually blocked out in some way with processed food. People are starving, bingeing, thinking about the next diet, wondering what excuses to make up for now *and* for later, wondering how much they weigh, or wondering how they can get some processed food or eat it without anyone noticing. This list is infinite. Denial may also go something like this:

"You say you're having difficulty losing weight?"
"Yes."
"Do you overeat a lot?"

"Not really. I have a [thyroid, hormonal, PCOS, emotional, etc.] problem."

"How much junk food do you ingest?"

"On the weekends, I'll go out with my friends and have some KFC or pizza."

"Have you ever binged on processed foods at all?"

"No, not really."

After I got to know this person, Karyn, and earned her trust, she shared with me one of her binges. This is what she had written in her food journal:

> *Thursday, it is 5:00 a.m. I just finished off a block of chocolate while watching TV, Smarties, a 200 g tub of yogurt, and Kingston cookies with ice cream. I then grazed for a while, which allowed me to do some work on the phone [I am in sales], grazing on a ripe pear; two Vita Brits, banana, sugar, and milk; two-and-a-half crumpets with butter and jam; and fatty chicken skin. Finally I went to bed, as I was feeling groggy, but I woke up a couple of hours later and ate M&Ms; gummy bears; two ham and chicken, tomato, cream cheese, butter sandwiches on multigrain; one slice of chocolate mud cake; one cherry ripe slice; one Snickers bar; two more slices of white bread and butter; rissoles; lamb chops (I only ate the fat tails off the chops) with fried egg, onions, grilled tomato; one scoop of chocolate chip ice cream; another cherry ripe slice; one peppermint Cornetto; potato chips ..."*

Karyn still didn't think she had a problem with processed foods. She thought she was the problem, because she couldn't control it like everyone else.

Joy gives another take on denial:

> *Call me whatever you want—anorexic, bulimic, emotional eater, compulsive overeater—but just don't call me a processed food addict. My father was an alcoholic; he was never home, and*

when he was, all he did was emotionally beat up on my mother. Then the physical abuse started. Mom took out a domestic violence order on him, as she was scared for us kids. There is no way, though, I am going to call myself an addict of any description. Plus, processed foods! Now come on! How can I be addicted to something that is legal to everyone at any age? I just have not been trying hard enough. Plus a friend of mine said she will help me this time to stay on my diet to lose this excess 26 lb. (12 kg.). That's all! I'm not as overweight as everyone else. On Monday, my friend Jo is coming with me to a new group to help me control the food and my weight.

There is no need to write any more about the denial stage of processed food addiction, as throughout this book, the message is quite clear. For the disease of addiction to stay active, there must be some sort of denial at play.

Anger

Anger is a necessary stage of the healing process. "I am angry I have this thing and I have tried everything to fix it, but nothing worked." The good news is there is nothing to fix. It is no one's fault that one is a processed food addict.

Be willing to feel your anger, even though it may seem endless. The more you truly feel it, the more it will begin to dissipate and the more you will heal. There are many other emotions under the anger, and you will get to them in time, but anger is the emotion we are most used to managing with ingesting processed foods.

Anger can be external or internal. I see patients with the disease of processed food addiction most typically turning their anger inwards, and I see quite a significant number of alcoholics in my clinic turning their anger outwards. I often wonder if this is gender related. No doubt some more research is needed down the road.

By keeping on ingesting the processed food or trying to control it, we are trying to keep the lid on our anger. Before we know it, we have several pots boiling on the stove, almost bubbling over. But hang on a minute—the processed food calls. We down some processed food and the pots go down to a simmer, until they get up to boiling point again. Each time we ingest processed food again, we are not dealing with the feelings, thoughts, and behaviors that are igniting our anger, or with the reality of an addiction diagnosis.

The truth is that anger has no limits. It can extend not only to yourself and your family but also to your friends, into work arenas, and even to health professionals. As I say to my patients, "You are not here to like me; you are here to get well."

Underneath anger is pain, your pain. It is natural to feel deserted and abandoned, and to feel that you still don't have your crutch—your coping substance. But we live in a society that fears anger. Anger is strength and it can be an anchor, giving temporary structure to the nothingness of the loss of an enemy or a friend in our endless supply of processed foods.

At first, grief feels like being lost at sea with no connection to anything. Then you get angry at someone, maybe a person who doesn't understand your disease of processed food addiction; maybe a person who isn't even around anymore because you're different since you accepted reality and you don't eat and drink like them now. Suddenly, you have a structure—your anger toward them. The anger becomes a bridge over the open sea, a connection from practicing your processed food addiction to recovering from it.

We usually know more about suppressing anger by stuffing processed foods down our throats than we do about feeling it. The anger is just another indication of the intensity of the malady, and by expressing it now, we don't have to ingest our anger anymore. Most importantly, we have our spiritual advisors, mentors, recovery buddies, addictionologists, and trained specialist addiction therapists to help us through our anger and this stage of recovery. Each day we don't ingest processed foods, our combined body, mind, and spirit learns how to cope with life without a substance.

Francine Shares About Anger

Why me?! I don't want this thing. I hate being a—whatever you call it—a processed food addict. I hate having to eliminate processed foods each and every day. I hate how my emotions are all coming up. Withdrawal sucks!! I just want to rip someone's head off. I'm scared my boss will fire me, as I've been quite short with clients of late. Even my partner is not liking this person he says I've become. He even said he preferred the old me, when I was ingesting processed foods, because at least he knew what to do.

Anger manifests differently in everyone, especially when we are withdrawing from processed foods. For the first time ever, we are feeling the feelings that were always stuffed down with processed foods. Anger can be quite scary in the early days; any feelings are threatening to the newly abstinent processed food addict. Indeed, when the disease was active (that is, when we were ingesting processed food), all our feelings were quite polarized. Happy or sad, good or bad, euphoric or depressed, fearful or in control.

Bargaining

Before experiencing the loss of something we have had or used for so long, it seems like we will do anything—if only we can ingest "the way I want, how I want, when I want, and weigh in at my desired weight."

"Please, God," we bargain, "this will be the last time I will ever ingest processed foods. *Tomorrow*, I promise, I will eliminate all processed foods, and I promise to never touch, buy, or ingest them again. If you just make my processed food addiction thing go away, I promise I will be good."

The disease of addiction is not about a person trying to be good, it is about a sick person trying to get well.

After we eliminate the processed foods, which feels like the biggest loss ever for us, bargaining may take the form of a temporary truce.

"What if I devote the rest of my life to helping others? Then can I wake up and realize this has all been a bad dream and be able to eat like a normal person and weigh in at my desired weight?"

We become lost in a maze of "if only this" or "what if that" statements. This can keep us in even more denial as we go about hooking in as many victims as we can to keep the disease operational. We want life returned to what it was; we want to keep our processed food and ingest it. We want to go back in time—see if we could have stopped earlier, or done something different, or recognized the symptoms of processed food addiction more quickly ... If only, if only, if only.

Guilt is often bargaining's companion. The *if onlys* cause us to find fault in ourselves and what we *think* we could have done differently. We may even bargain with the pain: "I won't put my fingers down my throat any more if ...." "I will lose weight now that it seems a bit more serious." "I will go to the gym no matter what!"

We will do anything not to have to change our lives; we just want this darn food problem thingy to go away.

Processed food addicts will change their circumstances and invent new ones, but changing themselves is out of the question. Most addicts are great at showing the world how they have everything together, other than "the food problem." But they reassure us that they are *onto* it, remaining in the past, trying to negotiate their way out of the hurt, the pain, the self-pity, the depression, the backaches, the dry mouth.

They keep doing the same thing over and over again, expecting a different result.

People often think of the stages of grief as lasting weeks or months. They may not realize that the stages are responses to feelings and behaviors that can last for minutes or hours or days or months, as they flip in and out of one stage of grief and into another. They do not enter and leave each individual stage in a linear fashion; they feel one, then another, and then go back again to the first stage, denial.

Penny Shares About Bargaining

> *When it comes to facing this disease, it was all about bargaining. I thought to myself, "Perhaps I've been bad. I promise I will be good now and never ingest again." I even bargained if God or whoever (I didn't care so long as it worked) could make me normal, then I would be the best mother, daughter, employer, employee, and more. I just wanted someone, something, or even this God to come down from wherever, tap me on the head, and make this all go away.*

I'm sure you have a bargaining story to share too. I look forward to hearing your shares.

Depression

After bargaining, our attention moves squarely to the present. A feeling of emptiness and hopelessness ensues, and grief enters our lives on a deeper level, deeper than we ever imagined. We learn that a lifestyle change is required. We learn new concepts, showing us how to put our life into our recovery, *not* our recovery into our life.

We ask ourselves, "Do I want this change? Am I capable of getting well? I feel just as bad now, feeling like this, as I did when I was ingesting (more than my share) of processed foods."

This depressive stage feels as though it will last forever. It's important to understand that this depression may not be a sign of mental illness but one of the myriad of consequences of addiction. It may also be comorbid; however, that is where the professional community comes in. If I am working with a patient for treating an addiction, I like to also incorporate other treatment staff, all of whom make decisions for the processed food addict until that person is able to think rationally and make personal decisions.

Sometimes, a patient may be unwilling to surrender, believing they can discern what is best for themselves, including whether or not they will carry on ingesting processed foods. That is to say, if the person refuses to accept the wisdom of the treatment team, they will generally ingest again. Sadly, society judges this person as being weak-willed or headstrong, but actually the addiction is controlling their actions and dominating their ability to make logical and rational decisions.

Thus, depression is an appropriate response in recovering from a disease—a disease that has ruled our lives for as long as we can remember. It feels like such a great loss. We withdraw from life, left in a fog of intense sadness, wondering perhaps if there is any point in going on alone. Why go on at all? Depression before, during, and after we eliminate processed foods is too often seen as unnatural: a state to be fixed, something to snap out of.

The first question to ask yourself is whether or not the situation you're in is actually depressing. The loss of my drug of choice—my beloved processed foods—feels like a very depressing situation. Depression is a normal and appropriate response. To not experience some level of depression after we eliminate processed foods would be unusual. Processed food was ingested by the processed food addict to help cope with life. Hence, learning to live without processed food while coming to the realization that we are processed food addicts, *and* accepting that we will never be able to ingest processed food like so-called normal people is understandably depressing, especially in the early days, weeks, and months of recovery. This is when the depression feels as though it will never end.

If grief is a process of healing, then depression is one of the many necessary steps along the way.

Amanda's Case Study

Amanda shared with me about her depression stage.

> *Depression, UGH!!! Every time I stopped ingesting processed foods I felt like s _ _ _ . I went to the doctors and told them how depressed I have been because of my yo-yoing weight—up and down, up and down, up and down. They gave me a script for some antidepressants and told me that should help with my depression. They didn't*

know how much I was ingesting. Of course, though, I wasn't going to tell them. Doc, if I wasn't so depressed, I would be able to lose the weight, then I wouldn't be so depressed about my life.

A penny for your thoughts. Do you identify with any or all of these stages thus far? You may like to share your story at www.addictionology.com.au.

Last but Definitely Not Least ... Acceptance

Acceptance is often confused with the notion of being "all right" or okay with what has happened. This is not the case here. Most people in early recovery find acceptance goes in and out as the rollercoaster of recovery takes over. The early elimination of processed foods (abstinence) is synonymous with a rollercoaster of emotions and moods. Progress and acceptance are tainted for a processed food addict in the early stages of recovery. They are new at feeling the reality of these emotions, which they are now discovering can change quickly from one moment to the next.

Until we can feel more at ease, until acceptance buries itself deep in our soul and we own our emotions, it will be much more challenging to move forward while cementing a daily plan for lifelong elimination of processed foods and recovery. I see acceptance when a patient finally stops fighting the diagnosis, that is, surrenders. I believe surrender—deeper surrender—continues each day the potential addict treats their disease. Their sense of self implies "everything is going to be okay." Therefore, this stage is about accepting the reality that we have a chronic disease and recognizing that this new reality is the permanent reality. We may take time to accept this reality or even to make it okay for now, but eventually we accept it. We learn to live with it. It is the new norm with which we must learn to live.

Chapter Six

Abstinence with Peace of Mind

*Abstinence
with peace of mind
is the norm
for a processed food addict.*

The Author

I coined the phrase "Abstinence—with peace of mind—is the norm for a processed food addict" several years ago, when I witnessed quite a few potential processed food addicts sharing that they were abstinent in other self-help groups but still felt restless, irritable, and discontented with their abstinence. As I listened to these individuals, they shared that a lot of their energy went into staying abstinent, with the underpinning message being "abstinence is all that is needed to lose weight." As such, this message and result shows whether they are in recovery or not.

Yes, indeed, we need to cut off the substance that is keeping the addiction alive. However, that in itself would not be enough to protect these individuals against their own biochemistry and the social pressure to ingest, as they learn to live a life without processed food.

For a processed food addict to recover, it is essential for them to learn and accept on a subliminal level that they are a real processed food addict, and any lurking notion or vision that somehow, someday, some way, they will be a normal eater has to be smashed.

Typically, chronic diseases require substantial lifestyle changes, and addiction is no different. Recovery is about implementing a new lifestyle. Over a period of time (this differs from one addict to the next, depending on their age and the severity of the disease), the processed food addict's body adapts to processed food, becoming more efficient at using processed food as its primary energy source. This enables the individual to function effectively even with a large volume of processed food in their system. This is why they suffer terribly when the processed food is eliminated—their body chemistry is in withdrawal from the primary substance it needed to go on living. Heightened depression, anxiety, stress, headaches, migraines, body aches, and pains are just a few of the symptoms experienced in the withdrawal process.

The processed food addict understands and accepts more and more the disease concept of addiction. For permanent recovery to take place one day at a time, they must learn how to live in a world without ingesting processed foods. Their disease of addiction is no longer operational. Thus, they need to mentally change their self-image, to picture themselves as an abstinent recovered processed food addict, with their beloved substance always missing.

Resisting this new norm at first, many potential processed food addicts want to maintain life as it was before they put the lid on the cookie jar for the last time. That is, they want to eliminate the substance without changing anything else, believing that they can still make all the decisions, including retaining the choice as to whether or not they will carry on ingesting processed food.

In time, though, through bits and pieces of acceptance, we see that we cannot maintain the past intact. It has been forever changed, and we learn to readjust. We learn to reorganize roles, reassign the things that made our lives unmanageable, and ask for help. We learn how to deal with each specific situation, rather than trying to do everything ourselves, as we don't have the processed foods to stuff down our thoughts and feelings and anesthetize our reality. Acceptance is realizing "Together we can; alone I'm gone!"

Finding acceptance may involve just having more good days than not-so-good ones. As we begin to live again and enjoy our life, we often feel that we are actually gaining a new freedom. We can never replace what has been lost by eliminating processed foods, but would we really want to keep the sleepless nights, the aches in our bodies, the mental torture of our minds? So, we make new connections, new meaningful relationships, new interdependencies.

Instead of denying our feelings, we listen to our needs: we move, we change, we grow, we evolve. We may start to reach out to others and become involved in their lives. We invest in our friendships and in our relationship with ourselves. We find ourselves being useful and purposeful, and we begin to live again. But we cannot do so until we have given grief its time for healing as we journey and take up our recovery path—it is ours for the taking.

Just one day at a time, we eliminate processed foods no matter what—this is the essence of acceptance, the beginning of a spiritual awakening and a life beyond our wildest dreams.

When I think of acceptance, it reminds me of when I was studying as an undergrad. I didn't want to go to university, much less do my first psychology degree. I had a world out there to live in. I too had just recovered from this malady. My dream was to be an air hostess, yet I found myself stuck in the back of a lecture hall, tears streaming down my face, trying to find ways to get me out of this place.

The tears, fears, and heartache continued at each lecture.

Then I started doing my honors, and I had a little bit more acceptance, but still I fought with it daily, weekly.

By the time I had come through my honors and completed my PhD, I decided it was pointless to fight this anymore. I accepted that this was my path in life and that I could fight it all I wanted, but I knew deep down it was pointless.

I must share that along the way I too had help from a lot of people, both professionals and laypeople. They have helped to keep me afloat over many years. You know who you are; unfortunately, many have passed away.

Today, I accept that this is my path and purpose in life, where I can be the most useful, in sharing, educating, researching, treating, and healing those suffering from this disease. Today, I continue to have a wonderful team around me who are the wind beneath my wings. As with addiction, we fight it, accept it a bit more, fight it, and accept it a bit more. I have found recovery is contagious. As Carl Jung said, "There is a strength in the protective wall of human community."

Case Study

Farrah shared with me about acceptance.

> *Acceptance of being a processed food addict always eluded me. Everyone else who was abstinent seemed to be able to accept this fact. I knew all there was to know; I read everything, listened to everyone, and then, finally, I realized I had tried everything known to mankind to beat this thing. Blessedly, it was pointed out to me that, as I went back through my eating career, I had been way out of control and didn't know it.*
>
> *I started to get help from a medical specialist trained in addiction diagnosis and treatment. He did a timeline of my disease, demonstrating the progression of my processed food addiction stages, highlighting to me just how processed food had dictated my life. I could see my job choices were all dictated by me being able to get to my one and only love!*
>
> *At school, my best friend's mother was the manager of the café. At the end of lunchtime, Lola and I would go to her mom and she would give us the leftover hot sausage rolls and caramel slices.*

When I was eighteen, I worked casually, which meant only five-hour shifts sometimes. This enabled me to finish work at 10:00 p.m. and call in to the late-night bakery that was open until midnight. I secured a full-time job at the local 7-Eleven. I was in heaven. I stacked all the shelves, especially around Christmas and Easter time, as any of the product that was damaged, I was allowed to eat and/or take home with me. Free food—yippee!

Then, through university, I knew all the food courts and food halls, who to eat with, when to eat, and when the best time was to show up—at closing time, of course, so I could buy all the processed food at one-third of the price, or if I was lucky, some bistros and diners gave away their leftovers.

Finally, graduating as a psychiatric nurse, I worked shift work and was well loved by everyone as I did the night shift. Well, this was just awesome. I got to graze all night, without anyone judging me.

At home, everyone was happy, as wife and mother was working. My friends did not judge me, because I was working; in fact, they were telling me how wonderful I was to do the shifts that no one else wanted. This went on and on.

Having the kids gave me even more alibis to stay overweight and in DENIAL. This just went on and on.

Seeing all this down on paper and listening to the doctor share about this disease, my denial started to be smashed. I finally eliminated processed food and accepted that there was nothing I could do about it other than to get help and treat it. What I believe helped me the most was the doctor reiterating quite a lot that the heart and soul of recovering from the disease of processed food addiction is accepting the disease concept of addiction.

There are many ways each individual accepts this disease. It doesn't matter how, when, or where they do. The main point is, they have. No one else can do this for you.

This is probably a good place to mention briefly the Serenity Prayer, which is well known in the recovery rooms of those who have recovered from addiction.

> *God grant me the serenity to accept the things I cannot change, Courage to change the things I can, And wisdom to know the difference.*
>
> *Reinhold Niebuhr (Rogers, 2005)*

In grieving, at times, some people will often report more stages or crossovers between stages. Grief is not linear; the stages all overlap as we experience a deeper acceptance. Hence, it is important to remember—*your grief* is as unique as you are.

CHAPTER SEVEN

Consequences of Processed Food Addiction

Withdrawal

The classic signs of any addiction are withdrawal and tolerance. What do these terms mean?

Let's start with *withdrawal*, which can be defined as "the development of physiological, psychological, and/or cognitive symptoms in response to periods of abstinence or reduced consumption of a substance" (APA, 2013). When the potential processed food addict suddenly reduces or ceases their ingestion of processed food, undesirable physical effects, coupled with unpleasant mood states, occur (e.g., irritability, anger, anxiety, skin irritations, etc.). Likewise, withdrawal can also mean ingesting more processed food to prevent these symptoms from arising.

Mary, a processed food addict in early recovery, shares that the physiological symptoms of withdrawal that "hammered" her included depression, anxiety, restlessness, discontentment, insomnia, restless leg syndrome, impulsively picking at her skin, disruptions to and absence of her menstrual cycle, and panic attacks.

Len reports being fidgety; having excruciating headaches, backaches, stomach aches, and pains; loneliness; and hot sweats, especially during the period straight after a binge. Len also suffered severe gout, from severe processed food addiction symptomology, and a heavy intake of alcohol, which exacerbated his withdrawal symptoms.

Jo shares that when she cuts back on cakes, pies, and baked goods, she feels light-headed and lethargic; these symptoms kick in even more after she has come through her first 24 to 72 hours of eliminating the processed foods.

Sometimes in the early stages of eliminating processed food, the processed food addict will consume massive amounts of coffee, consisting mainly of milk or cream. This leaves them feeling very agitated, with massive headaches and restlessness over the next week or two, and much longer for some people. Caffeine can be a processed food addict's go-to, as the caffeinated beverage can hijack the brain in the absence of the processed foods—but it will ultimately keep the craving active. This means even though they may be treating the disease by eliminating the primary substance, processed foods, they often continue to feel restless, irritable, and discontent (e.g., depressed, quick tempered, and hard to live with), as the combination of caffeine with milk or cream still sparks the craving.*

*Please note: The processed food addict is getting a kick not only from the coffee (caffeine) but also from the milk or cream (actually, the milk or cream provides the main kick). In the early days of detox, the addict will say, "I have not given up caffeine yet." However, it is not the caffeine the brain is chasing; it is the milk or cream that is doing the trick. The addict won't share anything about what they are adding to the coffee. This is another form of denial, and of keeping their addiction alive, so they are still getting some relief, until ... they ultimately ingest processed foods, again!

Beth Shares

> When I go on a diet, I drink more coffee; it helps to calm me down and enables me to at least function somewhat normally. Plus, it

> gets me through without bingeing, or at least it did in the early days. Actually, I have started to put a teaspoon of sweetener and a dash of skim milk in my coffee lately, which makes it taste even better. I also found that diet Coke and diet sodas helped me through the tough times. My newfound friends told me that the diet drinks may be free of sugar but the artificial sweeteners will spark off the craving. I thought I'd be fine, as I had six months under my belt by then and was in a routine of abstaining no matter what. Plus, I was going to anywhere between five and seven fellowship meetings a week (face-to-face meetings or phone meetings).
>
> Unfortunately, when I got to being abstinent for six months, I unintentionally picked up.

When Beth says she "picked up," it means she ingested processed food; it's similar to an alcoholic "falling off the wagon."

> I was at a food court with my best friend Jen and ordered a large coffee. She ordered a yogurt with dried fruit and nuts. She offered me some and would you believe I took it! It was only yogurt, dried fruit, and nuts! But then this, this ... craving ... started and before I knew it, I went back to the vendor and ordered some chocolate chip ice cream. I couldn't believe it.

Beth had all the support in the world around her, but she ingested again. What beat Beth back into the mire of processed food addiction? Was the addiction too strong in the end, or her psychological distress (depression, anxiety, and stress) too great? Was she a weak-willed glutton? Did she lack the self-discipline to say no at the food court? What finally made Beth ingest again?

One simple and quite astonishing explanation was that her caffeine and diet soda dependence, coupled with the extra non-processed foods she snuck in without telling anyone, kept the addiction simmering. Sometimes, Beth ate two cups of yogurt with a large bowl of blueberries and sweetener. Moreover, Beth drank caffeine at work, at home, with or without friends, and at some of her AA fellowship meetings. Sometimes she would swap to decaf (with sweetener and a large dash of milk), but she always ended up back at full strength, as it was the only thing that "settled" her.

Even though Beth presumably lasted (remained abstinent) for six months, she kept her disease of processed food addiction alive by still being intoxicated by the caffeine and the extra food, which played havoc with her blood glucose levels. Even though she wasn't ingesting sugar, flour, or wheat, the large consumption of non-processed foods, the caffeinated beverages, and the diet sodas she was drinking daily prevented her many interacting sick cells and organs from healing, so that her physiological systems could not get stronger and start to function normally.

Heavy loads of caffeine, diet beverages, and non-processed foods kept Beth's blood sugar unstable. It was only a matter of time before she craved the one substance she knew was the fastest way to *always* make her feel better—processed food. She wasn't eating the recommended amount of non-processed food (that is, just enough fuel for her body to function normally). Neither was she drinking enough healthy beverages to stabilize her blood glucose levels in order to make up for the decades of damage incurred while maintaining a high intake of processed foods and drinks. What Beth ate and drank confused her brain and fed her depression, anxiety, and stress while subliminally increasing her desire for processed foods. Ultimately, it made her abstinence a nightmare most days.

In summary, for Beth, eating insanely, plus caffeine and diet sodas, held her enslaved to her processed food addiction.

Many addicts supposedly in recovery are suffering like Beth and are in grave danger of a relapse. This isn't because they have no discipline or are in complete denial about their disease, but because they have not eliminated processed food, or are only tempering their processed food intake and other substances that can spark off the craving. Even their inclusion of high fat foods confuses the situation. They may be using caffeine, drinking diet sodas, eating three moderate meals a day, eating haphazardly, or eliminating sugar only. Blessedly, these processed food addicts may be spared much suffering of the withdrawal symptoms if they eliminate the substances that play havoc with their complex blood sugar chemistry.

Tolerance

Now let's briefly look at *tolerance*. Tolerance is a process whereby increasing amounts of processed food are required to achieve the former effects. For any potential processed food addict, the trick is to ingest (drink and/or use) to one's tolerance—that is, eat just enough processed food to prevent the withdrawal symptoms—and yet not ingest so much as to trigger the craving to binge more, vomit, lie on the couch, or be comatose later on. In other words, the trick is to try to be a functional processed food addict while still trying to control how much you ingest.

In the early stages of processed food addiction, trying to balance this act is not so challenging. However, the late-stage processed food addict will feel an overwhelming desire to ingest processed foods so they don't have to go through the torturous stages of withdrawal. But because they have a sickened (neurologically impaired) brain when it comes to ingesting processed foods, their judgment will be hindered as to how much is too much. As the disease of processed food addiction progresses, the margin of this balancing act narrows to a point where ingesting processed foods to a person's tolerance level is just a smidgen away from bingeing. As a result, obesity is the consequence, and/or more control methods are introduced with more bingeing periods.

The processed food addict is not ingesting because they are irresponsible, stubborn, undisciplined, or lacking in willpower—they continue to ingest processed foods because the disease has progressed, and their brains and bodies are no longer able to tolerate, cope, or function without having large amounts of processed foods in their system. Instilled in the memory of a processed food addict is the immediate comfort and benefits of ingesting, which blots out the knowledge of what will happen after ingesting. Moreover, always in the back of their mind is the hope that this time they can control it and get the great benefits they once did from ingesting. So, what seems absolutely necessary to the processed food addict occurs—they begin to ingest again!

You see, unbeknown to them, the processed food addict is chasing the effects that are similar to those obtained by using other substances, including satiety, a calmness of mind (to shut *the voice* up), and of course, the high. A feeling follows of being untouchable, with a new temporary mindset that they can now cope with anything and everything.

However, over time, the processed food addict finds there is a marked diminished effect, as she tries to keep her head above the water while ingesting the same amount. As we see in the shares below, a person's tolerance increases; that is, they need larger amounts of processed food to get the high—the anesthetization—from the processed food. Said in another way, the brain is hijacked by processed food and the individual (unbeknown to them) is under its influence. While the processed food addict has processed food in their system, they are able to function somewhat normally. They have developed a tolerance to the processed food and are now somewhat dependent on it. This potentially leads to progressing to the next stage of needing more and more processed foods in order to function.

Betty Shares

> *I would start out with a single Oreo, gradually increasing to several or a whole package of cookies. I used to be able to control it by only eating three cookies, but now I find I need more cookies to obtain that numbing-out feeling.*

Fiona Shares

> *I kept candies in the drawer at work. I started out eating only a handful at morning tea and afternoon tea time. Then I started*

> *having some before I started work, and then I'd stop off at the shops on the way home from work to get some of my favorites plus a few other goodies. It just got worse and worse.*

Leah Shares

> *When I used to buy the groceries, I would take them home, eat a snack, and get on with the rest of the day. But now I buy the groceries and I eat while lining up at the checkout. I make up excuses why I opened them before I bought them, such as I just found out I am pregnant and I need some sugar, or I am hypoglycemic, or I have a thyroid problem and I need to eat, or if I don't eat now my blood sugar will drop ...*

Annie Shares

> *I started off every day with a lovely cup of hot coffee. Then I went to a cappuccino, then added sweetener, then added a sugar, then two, and then more milk and less coffee ... Then I couldn't order the coffee unless I had it with a blueberry muffin, or two or three ...*

As the disease continues to progress, it leads to what is called *endurance*: "trying to endure the consequences of the last debacle." Eventually, a processed food addict finds that no matter how hard they try, they can't ingest processed foods 24-7. People need to sleep, work, attend to family commitments, and so on. Hence the processed food addict must endure withdrawal symptoms at some stage. Of course, the stronger the addiction, the worse the withdrawal symptoms; the worse the withdrawal symptoms, the further the disease is progressing; the further the disease is progressing, the more the processed food addict needs to ingest to numb out reality, or at least to try to function somewhat normally.

Simply said, a processed food addict needs to consume more and more of the processed foods in order to get the effect they crave to cope with life.

The processed food addict starts to conclude that they are weak-willed and pathetic, being blind to the fact that they are addicted to processed food. Or they are aware of their addiction but hope to overcome it through willpower. Over and over again, they fail in their efforts to stop ingesting processed foods or to temper their intake. This continual failure feeds their guilt, shame, and hopelessness.

"What is wrong with me? Why can't I stick to it? Why am I so weak?" they question themselves.

And of course, the ultimate question asked by every addict: "Why me?" The more they ingest, the more distressed they become because of the processed food's harmful effect on the brain.

As the saying goes in addiction circles, "A sick brain produces sick thoughts, and sick thoughts produce sick actions." In AA, it is often phrased as "Stinkin' thinkin' leads to drinkin'." A patient who was attending a 12-step-model PFA meeting shared the AA saying. I thought about this for a while and came up with "Rotten whingein' leads to bingein'."

While the processed food addict continues to try to endure, or moves to later phases of the addiction, the anguish and torment of withdrawal symptoms (known as *withdrawal syndrome*) can linger for weeks or even months in early abstinence. The longer the symptoms persist, the more exhausting and harder it is for the addict to stay away from processed food.

Heidi Shares

> *My disease of addiction makes me feel like I am sinking in a mire of quicksand, desperately trying to hold on to some tree branches but finding myself slipping inch by inch into the substance that I know is destroying me.*
>
> *I so desperately continue to hold on with every bit of willpower I can muster, but unfortunately, I keep being beaten by this persistent*

and overwhelming desire to ingest processed foods. I want to quit soooooo bad, but then I start to believe that I am better off when I am ingesting. At least I have the exquisite relief of the processed foods.

The Empty Processed Food Addict Syndrome

The Empty Processed Food Addict Syndrome

The Author

Just like a *dry drunk*, a processed food addict, whether ingesting or not, is still addicted to processed foods. "Once a processed food addict, always a processed food addict." If they only eliminate the substance—that is, processed foods—nothing else changes. This person is like someone whistling past the graveyard, trying to convince themselves they don't miss ingesting the processed foods at all. They may say they feel better, look better, perform their work better.

Unfortunately, I see this act all too often. The person is trying to convince themselves they are now fine, but deep down, they would do anything, or give anything, to eat a couple of bowls of ice cream (chocolate chip or cookies and cream, no doubt) and get away with it. Finally, it leads to taking that first bite (which they see others doing all around them). They are once again restless, irritable, and discontent—*and* most definitely not happy with their new lifestyle and abstinent way of living. To envision a life *without* processed foods to them is really worse than death.

At this stage, the processed food addict cannot live with processed food in their life or function without it. Living in a cloud of loneliness and isolation, the processed food addict will wish for the end. For them, not ingesting processed foods is akin to a death sentence. How does one come through this pain, this denial, this fear, this ... ad infinitum?

Kylie knows this place of despair only too well. She cannot imagine life *without* ingesting processed foods. She has controlled her ingestion for over nine months now. Her old life revolved around buying, eating, and getting rid of the processed food somehow, usually bingeing and purging up to three times a day. However, she saw and started to feel the toll this cycle was having on her body, mind, and spirit. She took between ten and forty laxatives after a binge and was a member of two 24-hour gyms, which allowed her to go to one gym at 2:00 a.m., when nobody else was there to judge her, and then attend the second gym during the day. She just wished she could be like other people.

The empty processed food addict can be under an illusion: "Now that I have my weight off or down to a certain goal weight, everything is and will continue to be fine."

A disease of addiction left untreated is a very sad state of affairs, not only for the processed food addict but also for those around her: spouses, partners, family, friends, colleagues! This person, if they are a *real* processed food addict, may participate in any number of controlling practices, but they will surely ingest again, sooner or later.

Controlling practices at this stage include the following:

- exercising as part of a guided fitness regime while adhering to a specific diet with other group members
- attending weight-loss groups
- attending diet clubs
- attending 12 step fellowship meetings for support and phoning a member every day to share what they will eat for that day
- just not ingesting processed foods

Unfortunately, and even worse, I believe, this person may continue to live wretchedly (miserably) being an empty processed food addict. Sadly, this is why some people who supposedly have several years (or decades) of abstinence and sustained weight loss but have changed nothing else wind up with a mental health diagnosis, are admitted to a mental health institution, or possibly die, without ingesting another single morsel of processed food.

Kylie Shares

> *My practicing days were like this: I would get up of a morning, go straight to the fridge, and pick up from where I'd left off the night before. Custard, leftover pizza, garlic bread, cheesecake. Then I would go back to the cupboard for chips, cookies, gummy bears, chocolate almonds, Toblerone ... I was in heaven—just me and my beloved processed foods.*
>
> *I got so full that I couldn't ingest another morsel. Panic would set in and the voice whispers would start. "You have to get rid of it NOW or you will be as big as a house." Off to the restroom, purge, and this relentless devastating process was repeated. However, over the last couple of years, I found I wasn't able to purge like I used to. Plus, my husband and friends were getting suspicious. Thank heavens I had the gyms and the laxatives as backups.*

Kylie sought help to enable her to control her ingestion of processed foods and its consequences—in particular, her weight—while also trying to control the subtle, inevitable insanity that precedes the first bite that sends her off again. Kylie knows a life without processed foods is daunting, fearsome, horrific. Sadly, she is dying a secret slow death.

As Kylie said many times, "K-L, this is hell. I can't do this, there is nothing I like that isn't processed. I just want to die."

Kylie attempts suicide, survives, and in desperation has a bit more of an open mind to learn how to live without her beloved friend, lover, enemy, her everything—her processed foods. She finally gives up hoping against hope this will be the last time. She makes a start to treat her disease of processed food addiction (submission). But eventually, the disease voice whispers sweet nothings in her ear, she leaves treatment, and after about three months, she goes back to her best friend. The devil she knows is better than the devil she doesn't, as life without her addiction was incomprehensible.

Let's have a look now at the difference between submission and surrender.

Submission Versus Surrender

Acceptance of any chronic illness is about understanding the disease and finding you have stopped fighting where you are at today. In the 12 step fellowships, the term *surrender* is repeatedly used. It simply means the processed food addict accepts they have the disease of addiction and is now willing to let go. This is understood as the person ceasing to hold on to their individual rigidities, with an ensuing sense of calm and acceptance that they have been beaten by processed food addiction. The core of this awareness is generally hopelessness and despair. In the act of surrendering, the person does not just admit defeat but accepts a power greater than themselves (which reduces the addict's ego), enabling the admission of much-needed outside help. This ego reduction is beneficial to the individual's personality makeup, because the processed food addict finally understands they have been suffering from a chronic illness that no amount of willpower can ever change.

In *submission*, the person does not really accept that they are unable to beat this chronic disease all by themselves, demonstrating that they are constantly struggling. *Submission* really only implies a passive cry, while the inner turmoil continues. Very few processed food addicts, active in the disease, can really comprehend how blind they are. Nor, as they start seeing glimpses of reality, can they endure this perception. A few will be inclined to label themselves *problem overeaters*, but they cannot bear the proposition that in reality they have a biochemical disease—that no amount of willpower will make them normal eaters. Their continual denial is backed by a universe that does not comprehend the difference between *sane eating* and *processed food addiction*.

Only when the person accepts on a subconscious level the reality of not being able to control and enjoy eating processed food like other people does the residual war stop. This is *surrender*. A sense of freedom is felt with knowing that the fight is finally over. Apart from a few fleeting moments of temptation, returning to ingesting processed food is implausible.

As with most diseases, our humanness may come into play in the years to come and we may think, "It would be nice to not have to weigh and measure, or be able to eat what I want, when I want, how I want, and where I want and be just like other people." However, if this kind of thinking does crop up, the processed food addict experiences a sense of great repulsion. Blessedly, they could not ingest the processed food even if they wanted to.

Once a processed food addict surrenders at the subconscious level, they will continue to receive messages at this subliminal level of the importance of and need for continued outside help for a prolonged or indefinite period of time. They will be in the possession of a newfound peace and sincerity that will pave the way for continued constructive action, taking the place of the shallow assurances of merely conforming temporarily until once again the memory of their suffering and self-pity weakens, and their need to comply lessens.

Multi-comorbidity

Comorbidity and *multi-comorbidity* are medical terms referring to the presence of one or more additional conditions or diseases co-occurring with a primary condition in the same person at the same time.

Many individuals with an addiction have a coexisting mental health condition, for example, bipolar disorder.

An addict may ask herself, "Do I eliminate all my potential addictive substances *in one go*? Alcohol, drugs (over the counter, prescription, or illicit), nicotine, pills, caffeine, and processed food?"

Franny, another patient, works at a well-known IT company and appears to be functioning at work. She has eliminated nicotine, drugs, and alcohol but suspects she has a problem with processed foods. Franny has been able to stay sober for long periods of time with the help of nicotine and processed foods, but she has relapsed into alcohol use after first six years and then eight years of sobriety.

She blamed her circumstances—her husband started drinking again and work was not all that great, therefore she had no money to feed her addiction. In reality, Franny has just swapped the witch for the bitch, that is, put one substance down but kept her brain happy with other substances. Meanwhile, her blood sugar is very unstable, producing roller-coaster mood swings. Indeed, all these issues didn't help Franny stay sober, as her brain was still being hijacked by another substance.

If nothing changes, nothing changes.

I have found it best to deal with one addiction at a time. Fortunately, a number of patients have already eliminated the alcohol, nicotine, and drugs with professional help before coming to me. Plus they regularly attend the self-help groups of Alcoholics Anonymous and Narcotics Anonymous. And then they find the weight piles on and start to look at the possibility of processed food addiction. It is quite common to see alcohol eliminated first, followed by nicotine, gambling and/or drugs, with the last to be eliminated being processed food. Of course, this isn't the same for everyone, as each addiction manifests differently in each person. The saying "first things first" sums this up for me in a nutshell.

CHAPTER EIGHT

Changing Addiction Diagnoses and Treatments

I believe diagnosis and treatment of addiction will change over the next ten years. Take for example alcoholism. In the past, if an individual presented with alcoholic symptomology, then they would be diagnosed and treated for alcoholism—that is, they would be treated for the substance, alcohol. Today and moving forward, I see professionals working in the field of addiction medicine will begin to understand the disease of addiction in *its entirety* and so primarily and routinely treat *the disease of addiction* and not just *a* or *the* substance.

Many recovering alcoholics, drug addicts, and the like are still suffering—just staving off a relapse—not because they have no willpower or are continually kidding themselves about their *problem*, but because the craving for the primary substance is being kept alive with one or more still-active addictions. The mood swings, restlessness, irritability, and discontentedness are the result of the addict's body chemistry gone awry. The individual with the addiction does not understand what it means to be afflicted with this disease. High relapse symptoms are born from ignorance—not understanding the biochemical makeup of the addiction—which leads to addicts not knowing how to keep their disease in remission and safeguard themselves against it.

I believe striving for permanent recovery, one day at a time, is what counts in addiction treatment.

A Family Disease

Processed food addiction is a family disease. It requires the family to recover.

An important point to reiterate is that a family member, partner, or significant other has the key to free the addict from her addiction. While the partner may be enabling the addict (that is, taking away all the evidence and aftermath of the disease and not allowing the addict to take responsibility for the consequences of ingesting processed foods), they too are on a roundabout of denial. As they continue to struggle to try to fix the addict, they are actually keeping the addiction alive.

More often than not, it is at this stage that recovery can be initiated by the decisions and actions of loved ones, friends, family, employers, and employees, and even those from the helping professions, for that matter. These enablers—let's call them *the players*—in their various forms have the key to unlock the processed food addict's denial and therefore to start them down the road of recovery. At this stage, it is important that those in the processed food addict's life learn how different people affect each other in keeping this disease operational; then they can commence to learn the most challenging part of all: a way of life that is completely alternative to what they have been doing in the past.

The processed food addict is locked in by their illness. Fortunately, the players, in quite a lot of cases, hold the key to the lock—the addict's first step to freedom.

In the beginning, this can be quite challenging for the significant other, family members, friends, and colleagues of the processed food addict, and they may find they are standing alone. Others around the addict may think these players are deserting this helpless person, especially if there are no other substitutes to take on the old role of enabling the processed food addict.

I can assure you, the processed food addict will be extremely angry when this person, the enabler, does *not* do as they wish. More often than not, what keeps the processed food addict in denial is the mistaken belief that the enabler (spouse, partner, friend) wants to learn how to stop them from ingesting processed foods, so they can *fix* their loved one. Unfortunately, this only keeps the disease in denial and allows the processed food addict to continue believing that nothing is wrong with them—they are just fine, thank you. Above all, they will go to any lengths to make sure no one meddles in anything to do with how much they ingest and the subsequent consequences, but the enabler had better be there to pick up the pieces once again. In the processed food addict's mind, she is right and everybody else is wrong; she only needs to try just one more diet, gym, nutritionist, clinician, self-help book, ad nauseam. I often say to patients, "A processed food addict can sell ice to an Eskimo today and turn around and sell ice to the same Eskimo tomorrow for double the price."

Back in the day when AA's 12 step program was in its embryonic stage, a number of medical clinicians, including psychologists and doctors, investigated a sampling of problem drinkers. Their aim was to discern what personality characteristics these individuals had in common. Results highlighted that the majority of the participants being examined were still immature, emotionally sensitive, and grandiose (*Alcoholics Anonymous*, 1988). This, I believe, still rings true today when I meet a typical processed food addict for the first time.

A potential processed food addict may weigh 240 lb. (109 kg.) and be living to eat (not eating to live), or they may weigh 90 lb. (41 kg.) but be purging three times a day. If you ask them how much they have eaten on a daily basis over the past week or two, their answer will be anything *but* the truth. The processed food addict will do anything to stay in control of everyone and everything, as they themselves do not know when that mental twist, so subtly powerful, will haunt them again. It is a force so compelling that in order to obey its demands, they always have to be prepared.

That reminds me of a patient who, when first starting to eliminate processed foods, was so frightened of the "robotic desire to ingest" (as she described her powerlessness) that she always carried an extra couple of dollars in her bag. That way, she could buy a chocolate bar or some cookies to subdue a craving just in case the mental obsession to eat kicked in.

Of course, it wouldn't buy much these days, but when the phenomenon of craving kicks in, a few candies or cookies may be enough to tide the addict over until they get to the real binge, which is where they are heading to next. After a binge, they once again awaken and are sickened by what they vaguely remember. These memories are like a traumatic dream, and the processed food addict continues to feel extremely tense with the thought that someone might have seen them. Primarily, they try to subdue these feelings, hoping they will never resurface, which naturally leaves the addict under severe psychological distress—a distress that, of course, only more processed foods will alleviate ... for the time being. There is no easy, soft way to stop a roundabout of denial. Those on it, spinning around and around, believe it is much more painful to stop than to keep it spinning. Change, at the best of times, is a frightening proposition.

As I have said, the disease of processed food addiction manifests differently in each individual; hence, it is challenging to follow specific rules intended for every person suffering from the disease. Even though each scenario is different, the framework of the roundabout of denial remains the same. The most challenging concept in halting the repeating cycles is the high anxiety and associated fears that the processed food addict won't make it without the help of a significant other (enabler in various forms). The enabler thinks they are helping. Unfortunately—unbeknown to them—their help actually permits the addict to continue to ingest processed foods and to use the enabler as the perfect remedy for all their problems with life.

A book of recovery for the family of a processed food addict is outside the scope of this writing; however, a professional who has processed food addicts or their family members as patients or clients can guide the persons involved in learning to cope with processed food addiction without enabling the addict.

Intervention

Learning and understanding more about the disease of addiction is the foundation of treatment ... and establishing a lifelong recovery program. By the time a processed food addict starts getting serious about wanting to recover, they have tried everything else—weight-loss groups, self-help groups (12 step food programs), exercise, psychological approaches, even weight-loss surgery. And the list goes on. As the processed food addict continues to learn about their illness, they will come to understand they are powerless over their illness, and why they are among a specific group of people who cannot ingest processed foods in the way everyone else appears to.

I am actually not as quick these days to commit to that last statement wholeheartedly, as every second person says they have an allergy to something. However, as with any illness, explanations are a must for the individual to comprehend what is actually happening to them and, more importantly, to help them understand and appreciate what it will take to get well and stay well. When the processed food addict knows better, they can learn the wisdom to do better, as nothing wards off temptation better than being proactive in learning and taking action to implement a recovery treatment program. Therefore, adjusting to this new way of living that does not include processed foods in turn cements a new lifestyle that will protect their recovery, keeping the disease of addiction in remission one day at a time.

There are several strategies to consider when recovering from processed food addiction.

1. Spiritual Insight

The first strategy to consider is to gain spiritual insight. That is, to start with self-honesty, open-mindedness, and a willingness to get well. Continued patience, persistence, and perseverance in learning and understanding, through various means, the exact nature of processed food addiction in one's own life sets up a foundation for smashing the denial of previous years or decades.

A large number of processed food addicts come from dysfunctional homes. Effective treatment can sort through the unmanageability of their lives, previously dictated by processed foods, and begin to construct a new way of living. This would include understanding the following:

- how the disease of processed food addiction develops and progresses over time
- why the processed food addict cannot safely ingest one crumb of processed food ever again
- why the processed food addict experiences a sudden urge to ingest processed foods
- why processed foods make them feel better
- why the processed food addict suffers psychological distress (depression, anxiety, and stress) when they stop ingesting processed foods
- how processed food addiction has affected their brain (neurological pathways), behavior, and personality
- why the processed food addict will most definitely return to ingesting processed foods if their disease is not treated (relapse)

As with all chronic diseases, before any treatment can be implemented and sustained, the person with the symptoms must understand what their diagnosis is, what it means, and what happens next.

Let's use an example of a person with type 2 diabetes (t2d). Many questions come into play in the important early stages of diagnosis and treatment: "How did I get to be diagnosed with t2d? Is it hereditary? No one in my family appears to have had it or got it now. Will I be on medication for the rest of my life? Will it progress? How do I tell my family? I'm scared it will change everything in my life. How will I and my family cope? What about my work, how will it be affected? I have plans to go on an overseas vacation; how do I watch my blood sugar while I am away?"

These questions and many more like them are very pertinent in the early stages of treatment among people with t2d. That is why a professional endocrinologist who has had experience in diagnosing, treating, and stabilizing the disease is of the utmost importance. Chronic diseases are life-threatening! A diabetes caregiver or health nurse may be able to help the individual with their diabetes care plan in the early days, but if the diagnosis is severe, then a professional must be sought.

Similar questions arise for someone with a potential processed food addiction diagnosis. "Why me? Why am I *an addict*, let alone a processed food addict? My aunt Emily was morbidly overweight, but she is now eighty and she seems to have gotten by. How will I live without it? Everywhere you look, there is processed food. What about my work? I have plans to go on a cruise in eight weeks' time; it will be no fun if I can't eat at the all-inclusive buffet."

These and many similar questions arise, as the disease diagnosis may be the same, but the illness is multifactorial, manifesting differently in each case. That is why a professional such as an addictionologist, addictionist, or an accredited addictions therapist who has had experience in addiction—from diagnosis to treatment—must be sought. Helping individuals understand their disease and what they have to do to keep the disease in remission one day at a time is paramount.

Just to reiterate: not everyone who eats processed foods is a processed food addict, just as not everyone who eats has t2d. Some potential processed food addicts may have prediabetes, and some may not cross the physiological line to dependence.

Clinicians who specialize in treating other manifestations of disordered eating (including binge eating disorder [BED], anorexia, and bulimia) abound these days. While these behavioral and/or psychological approaches may be of great benefit to the majority of people with disordered eating issues, weight problems, and the like, I have found that once a person is a processed food addict, they are always a processed food addict.

Over time, the disease of processed food addiction progresses. Treating fluctuations in weight (gains or losses), malnutrition, unhappiness (known also as *anhedonia*), insomnia, depression, anxiety, stress, grief, shame, isolation, low self-esteem, backaches, joint pain, migraines, and the like will not touch the addiction. This is perhaps why other methods have failed entirely, because treating the symptoms of the disease does not touch the primary cause—processed food addiction.

2. Nutritional Hygiene

Learning about nutritional hygiene is the second step. By weighing the non-processed foods we ingest, we are automatically implementing a regime to eliminate processed foods and the overall volume of food intake. Additionally, taking vitamins and minerals allows a processed food addict's internal organs to regenerate while repairing damaged cells, building the immune system, and bolstering the processed food addict's defenses against other ailments. Furthermore, having plenty of rest and commencing to exercise are invaluable in the early days, weeks, or months, while the body is going through the withdrawal stages.

Ideally, rest and exercise will become a natural coping mechanism later on when dealing with life on life's terms. With nutritional hygiene, the processed food addiction will remain in remission, creating less of a threat that the craving of processed foods will reawaken the allergy that plagues so many processed food addicts long after their last bite.

3. Self-Help Group

A self-help group creates a protective wall of human community. The 12 step model of AA is the most tried and proven method globally for helping alcoholics stay sober. Therefore a 12 step framework (based solely on the 12 steps, 12 traditions, and 12 concepts of AA) is implemented in treating the disease of processed food addiction.

A support group is essential because its members are dedicated to supporting each other in the continual elimination of processed foods on a daily basis.

Taking pains to abide by the principles of AA, Processed Food Anonymous (PFA) helps processed food addicts recognize they are licked by their disease of processed food addiction and powerless to fight it on their own.

As the processed food addict is healing, the 12 step fellowship provides identification and support in an environment with other abstinent processed food addicts.

- Belonging to such a fellowship helps to reiterate the disease concept of addiction—the processed food addict comes to understand they are primarily recovering from a disease—not from symptoms of disordered eating (symptoms such as weight).
- Additionally, the processed food addict learns to grow up, coupled with new living skills that were negated while ingesting processed foods. They learn how to increase their self-esteem, relate to each other, deal with success and failure, cooperate, and listen. They basically learn how to deal with life's up and downs ... all without the use of a substance.

- Processed Food Anonymous's foundation lies in cutting off the source of the trouble—processed foods—while eliminating dependence on people, places, and things; and in learning how to rely on a strength and power greater than oneself to solve the problem—processed food addiction.

A Threefold Disease

What does it mean when we say addiction is a threefold disease?

Recovery from a processed food addiction, like recovery from other substance addictions, comprises three areas of recovery. In the early years of AA, and likewise today, addiction was recognized as a threefold disease: physical, mental, and spiritual (*Alcoholics Anonymous*, 1939).

I will cover the physical and mental recoveries first. Further down, I'll cover the spiritual recovery.

Physical

The consumption of processed foods by processed food addicts is a manifestation of an allergy—a physical craving by the body to want to ingest more and more, even if the person is so full they cannot possibly do so. This is similar to an alcoholic who has an allergy for alcohol; one is too many and a hundred are not enough. Once the alcoholic drinks the alcohol, they spark off a phenomenon of craving. The late Dr. William D. Silkworth's theory of alcoholism states, "the body of the alcoholic is quite as abnormal as his mind" (p. xxiv, *Alcoholics Anonymous*, 1939). Silkworth went on to explain that the action of alcohol on chronic alcoholics is a manifestation of an allergy, that the phenomenon of craving is limited to this class and never occurs in the average temperate drinker, and that these allergic types can never safely use alcohol in any form at all. Moreover, Silkworth's statement implies that in certain alcohol abusers psychological approaches were futile and that when treating alcoholism, it is imperative to treat the physical factor (the body) of the addiction in addition to the abnormality of the mind.

This is the same for the processed food addict. That is, ingesting processed food makes them feel better, and they "need it to function." In their mind, processed food will fix everything. It is a blessing, not a curse; it is their antidote, not their poison. For a brief period of time (which shortens as the disease of addiction progresses), ingesting processed food floats away their worries, their fears seem to evaporate, their psychological distress diminishes, and loneliness is no more. This appears to solve all their problems.

Such an addiction is like a default mechanism that only occurs among certain individuals. As life becomes too much to deal with throughout the day, they reach out for the only known perfect elixir. Succumbing to the craving again, as they have many, many times before, their allergy kicks in, and before they know it, they are in the familiar phases of intoxication. They surface with the relentless withdrawal symptoms and vow to never ingest processed foods again.

If someone is allergic to strawberries, they will break out in a rash. If they have a dairy allergy, they will get diarrhea. Many people in today's society have an allergy to peanuts, which causes severe reactions and can be fatal.

The processed food addict's allergy, which is similar to an alcoholic's allergy, manifests when they introduce a crumb of processed food into their system, setting off an uncontrollable craving (the allergy) to ingest more and more. Said in another way, when a processed food addict ingests processed food, the manifestation of their allergy is a craving of the body to ingest more and more and more. Once the food is ingested, this allergy will kick in under any and all circumstances, no matter whoever, whatever, or wherever. The addict has to physically keep consuming the substance. This allergy is what sets the processed food addict apart from other people, who are able to control and enjoy their intake of processed foods without any repercussions. The substance, processed food, also melts away the addict's fears, loneliness, depression, anxiety, and stress, and solves *all* their problems—one of their problems being the promise that they can ingest all the processed foods they want now, as this time it will be different. Hence, they pass into the well-known stages of a binge, swearing never to do that again and promising that tomorrow (preferably Monday) they will start a new diet, the diet that will end all diets and *fix* them.

Olivia Shares

I have been to this place many times before. I can be on a diet (which is the diet to end all diets, of course) and then for some reason or another, I ingest a morsel of processed foods and then I can't stop. I tell myself, "I will just have this and that and stop when I get home." I get home, and then I'm in the kitchen trying to make the microwave shut up, so its beep doesn't wake my boyfriend. I'm feeling like a failure again ... Then I ask myself how did I get started again ... ?

Sometimes I don't even need a reason, for that matter. I may not even be thinking about ingesting processed foods, then all of a sudden this thought enters my head and says, "I have been so good for the past six weeks. I have lost 7 kilograms, one something-or-other won't hurt me. I deserve it."

Mia Shares

The best way I can describe it is, it's like a light switch, as if someone flicks on a switch in my brain and then before I know it, I ingest just one bite of a slice of garlic bread and I'm off again—a whole pizza, frozen Coke, and two chocolate mousses later.

It is impossible for me to turn the light switch back off.

What I find to be the worst part about all this is, when I try and tell someone (family, best friends, doctors), they just don't get it. They then tell me to do this or do that. I think to myself, "If I could darn well (expletive) do that, don't you think I would!"

Being a recovered processed food addict today, I now realize that not everyone is going to understand. It took me quite a few decades (I am now in my forties) to comprehend what the truth was for me. Paradoxically, when I started to get well, treat my disease, and not care what others thought, others seemed to automatically support me. Not so much understand, but they just accepted me as Mia.

This is what I have to do today to stay well. The light switch has been turned off and the negative voice does not whisper today about processed foods, which is the biggest miracle of my life. The only way I can describe it is, I feel like someone has treated me for another chronic disease such as cancer, and now it is in remission.

Mental

The mental condition of a practicing processed food addict is distorted, and the majority of processed food addicts cannot stay abstinent in the early days without help. Several find it challenging but are able to stay abstinent for a short period of time, but weeks or months later they find themselves staring into the face of an alive, irresistible need to ingest processed foods.

Some patients describe this need (the phenomenon of craving) as if it is animated, a real presence, and its force is so compelling that it seems to be external to the processed food addict. Furthermore, this phenomenon of craving appears to be limited to this class of people and never occurs in the majority of people who may be dieting today or eating what and when they want.

What is consistent in clinic is that these allergic types can never safely ingest processed foods without sparking off that phenomenon of craving. Once processed food is ingested in any form at all, they have an inability to stop, no matter how much they may want to. Like the alcoholic, if they do succumb once again (which is typical), they find that no matter what they do, they cannot stop the phenomenon of craving that becomes the overriding force in their lives.

A processed food addict may go on more diets; try more weight-loss plans; join gyms; study nutrition, naturopathy, psychology, medicine, or law; get their jaws wired or their stomachs stapled (weight-loss surgery); undergo cognitive behavior therapy; or take mindfulness courses in order to control this craving. However, they find that each time they try something new or different (which may last a couple of days or weeks or, if they are lucky, longer), it is even harder to moderate or stop altogether than the last time. Ultimately, processed food addiction is a progressive, chronic disease—it gets worse over a period of time, never better.

Indeed, if the disease were just physiological, it would stand to reason that if the person never ingested processed foods—sparking off the phenomenon of craving and setting the addictive cycle in motion—then that would be the end of the story. Researchers over the decades have investigated methods of dieting and implementing healthy lifestyles to try to stop, moderate, or cut down an individual's junk food intake. These included changing the person's actions and behaviors (e.g., not walking past the local takeout joints or bakeries where they usually binged), writing affirmations and using subliminal tapes to reiterate "I won't ingest processed food for the next 24 hours," and phoning another person every day (sometimes six times a day) to stop from ingesting processed food. Unfortunately, these methods do not work over a long period of time if someone is a severe processed food addict.

Although there are a number of people who have made some headway through psychological, psychiatric, or surgical approaches, in the larger scheme of things there is still a proportion of people who do not respond to these approaches. Professionally, as someone who treats processed food addiction on the job day in and day out and empathizes with the totality of destruction that comes with addiction—including the loss of family, jobs, and friends, not to mention the increasing secondary complications of obesity, t2d, hypertension, cardiac disease, joint and bone disease, stroke, and sleep apnea—I cannot but encourage others to realize that the treatment of processed food addiction is analogous to the treatment of other addictive substances. I find each day I treat another processed food addict, I become more aware that a number of people who are real processed food addicts do not respond to the typical psychiatric, psychological, and surgical methods available in today's society. They are the ones who are allergic to processed food.

Joanna Shares

> I knew I had a problem with ingesting sugar, flour, and wheat, but so did some other people I was hanging around with. Yet they seemed to be doing okay.

> I learned a bit about food addiction, and a doctor suggested that I might be a bit worse than I actually thought. Moreover, she said that if I had a real processed food addict mindset, then sooner or later, I would ingest again over something very trivial, even against my own will not to.

> I told her that the others were doing fine and I too just needed to be able to control the volumizing on non-processed foods, cut back the six to eight cans of diet soda I was drinking, as well as eliminate the nuts and dried fruit, and then I too would get it. Others seemed to be able to do it.

> I had heard of processed food addiction but didn't think I was that far gone, and I thought that really those others were just doing what I was doing anyway, and more than likely, the doctor was making a mountain out of a molehill.

Joanna believed she could get by just like the others and temper her ingestion of food. However, she did *pick up* her addiction several times in succession. Here is her account of her last spree.

> I was finally doing well. I had been abstinent for approximately eight months and was holding on to a 55-lb. (25-kg.) weight loss. I was meeting my mother to look for a flat iron for my hair.

We sat down at the food court and I pulled out my abstinent lunch loaf. Mom was used to how I ate. I actually enjoyed my non-processed food meals. My feet were tired. Moreover, I felt tired because Mom could be a little overbearing at times, as she was quite elderly. But I thought I was being good to invite her, being a dutiful daughter and all.

As I finished off my lunch, I thought of how much Mom loved cappuccino, so I decided to get her one. But then this thought crossed my mind that one wouldn't hurt me either, as I had already eaten my abstinent lunch. So, I ordered one for Mom and one for me too.

Something didn't feel right, but since I was having it with my meal and being sociable with Mom, it would be fine. Ahh ... it tasted like heaven. What came with it, though, was a miniature cookie. I quickly downed it too, as it was part of the coffee deal I had paid for. I didn't even think before I ingested the cookie. I then ordered another one while Mom was finishing off hers. As we got up to leave, I decided that perhaps I was making too big a deal of things, so I ordered a package of cookies like the one that came with my coffee to have when I got home ...

Consequently, I ended up bingeing that evening, and found myself the next day not being able to face myself or my work, so I didn't go to work. The headaches came back in an instant, I started picking at my sores and eating the scabs again, my back ached from the amount of processed food I ingested, and this negative voice characteristic of this devilish addict personality would not shut up. It was relentless. "Why did you do it again? You knew better than that! No one will love you if you put on weight and are fat. You have just gained 6 lb. (3 kg.). You are so weak-willed, just a hopeless case!"

Even though Joanna knew about food addiction, and knew that she might be a real processed food addict after all, she thought if she just did certain things that others were doing, she would be fixed and would be able to maintain her weight loss. Though conscious of the fact that she might one day give in to an imperious urge, Joanna thought she would be fine and it wasn't that bad. However, all the things she had learned did not even come into play. Her mind was so powerful that there were *no* other options but to pick up.

Most folks call this plain insanity. Sure, she ingested a cup of coffee and a cookie—why didn't she stop then? She had just lost all that weight. Why would she be so foolish and put herself at risk of gaining it back again?

For practicing processed food addicts, this type of thinking is the norm. The insanity is that the processed food addict keeps doing it over and over again and can't stop. As the saying goes, the definition of insanity is doing the same things over and over again and expecting a different result. Even when some addicts reflect on the consequences of ingesting, that thought is overridden by more crazy thinking, rationalizing "just one won't hurt me."

Amelia Shares

> *I thought self-knowledge would fix me. I went to numerous workshops on food addiction and learned about relapsing and some good information about the brain.*
>
> *As I contemplated my history and memberships and attendances at ALL the well-known weight-loss groups, and a myriad of other ventures, I decided there was no way I would pick up again.*
>
> *I was now a successful teacher. In just nine months and after losing quite a lot of weight, I was promoted to Head of the Home Economics Department.*
>
> *I stayed empty from those foods suggested by my self-help group—mainly sugar, but also flour and wheat were mentioned a lot. I was warned that I may be suffering from a mental obsession so*

> *profoundly powerful that it would, sooner or later, blindly take over and I would start to ingest processed foods again.*
>
> *"How could this be possible?" I thought. I was head of the department, I had lost 60 lb. (27 kg.), I was in a new relationship, and I had built up plenty of support around me. With willpower.*

Amelia thought willpower would help her to stay vigilant and strong.

She had no problem declining the pre-dinner goodies when she went out, the cocktails, canapés, and entrées that came her way. At lunchtime in the staff room, everyone encouraged her to keep going and admired her strong willpower, wishing they could be like her. A couple of months later, she went to a school reunion back in her hometown. She was so excited, as she had not seen some of these friends since her school days; the ones she had seen only remembered her as being overweight.

> *Attending the reunion, I was so excited to see everyone and loved the compliments I was receiving on how good I was now looking, not to mention how successful I was becoming with my teaching career. Just as I came out of the restroom, a waiter offered me a mini quiche. The thought crossed my mind that one quiche (no more) wouldn't hurt, as I would be having my abstinent meal that I had prepared the night before, so all would be well.*
>
> *Ahh ... the quiche tasted divine. So I caught the waiter's eye and took another one. It was time to sit down for dinner. As planned, the waiter brought out my pre-cooked meal, now beautifully presented on their dinnerware. After dinner, the music began, and I danced the night away.*
>
> *I started heading to my hotel room when it hit me. I had been dancing and burning up heaps of calories. I even missed the dessert servings, so I thought I had better order something light from room service, and I did. I not only ordered something light but I remembered there was a vending machine just down the hall from*

my room; it sold chips and chocolate bars. So, I headed down the corridor.

The next morning, I woke up feeling—to be honest, I don't know how to describe my feelings that next morning. No words could really explain the depth of despair, depression, fear, worry, hopelessness, and unworthiness that were flowing through my body, mind, and spirit.

I remembered the forewarnings that if I was a real processed food addict, a time and day would come when I wouldn't have any willpower against the first bite of processed food. I now know that I am a real processed food addict, and I can empathize with people who share that a problem had them hopelessly beaten. The notion that I could be like those who still have a tiny margin of control was smashed.

The illness of processed food addiction starts off in the mind and not the body. If asked "Why on earth did you pick up again and get wasted, especially when you know what it does to you?," most processed food addicts, in all probability, will give you a million reasons, coupled with an extensive list of alibis, why they did it, again. Or they will become anxious and not respond, or change the subject.

In reality, they are just as confused as you are about why they picked up again. They may share a little bit about what happened, but if they are honest with themselves, they are just as baffled as everyone else as to why they did it, again. Deep down in their heart of hearts, they too can't understand their craziness.

By this time, those around the processed food addict believe that what she does is not the norm, but they still hope and pray she will wake up one day as if she had been in a bad dream and assert a level of control just like everyone else.

This is where the processed food addict crosses the line to physiological dependency. At a certain point, the processed food addict has tried every conceivable remedy to fix their condition. Even though they may have the strongest willpower coupled with a mighty urge to stop ingesting processed foods, they still cannot stop. This is analogous to other people who deal with chronic diseases on a daily basis. Their illness may go into remission, but they won't be able to fix it by their own willpower.

A person with cardiac disease cannot attain enough stamina to run a marathon, just as a person with diabetes cannot drum up enough willpower to think down their blood glucose levels. The addict is like a person who has lost a limb; it is impossible to grow another limb.

In the early years of treating this disease, I too tried to help a person ingest processed foods normally, but after a couple of clinic hours, I knew processed food addiction was at play, and I have never been able to produce a normal eater out of a processed food addict and never will.

Blessedly, I know my limits. Maybe one day evolving systematic enterprises of the twenty-first century that investigate and test new products and procedures, or explanations and predictions about processed food addiction, will be successful. However, it has not been the case for many, many, many decades.

A Devilish Alter Ego: The Ignoble Personality of Addiction

I have discussed in the preceding pages the ignoble and bestial character, the negative mind, the negative self-talker, the second self, the disease voice, the devilish alter ego, the addict personality—a gremlin that lurks in the network of one's mind and disguises itself, sending never-ending rhetorical messages in all phases of processed food abuse.

In the early days of AA, a book titled *Our Devilish Alcoholic Personalities* was dedicated to the members of AA globally. This personality, known as *odap*, was characterized as an antagonistic little mental monkey that lured AA members, using its rhetorical voice to whisper destructive, anti-sober temptations (Webster, 1970). Please note, I have purposely written *odap* in lowercase to express the toxic, lower nature of the disease in processed food addiction.

In clinic, processed food addicts start out with the recognition of their bestial and ignoble *devilish addict personality*. In the early days of treatment, my patient and I will name this voice, which is personal to the individual at the time. I have come across some interesting names over the years; my favorite is *fos*, which stood for "full of sh*t." The processed food addict believed that every time this voice spoke it was "full of sh*t"! Another was *pita*, for "pain in the ass." There was also *Ms. Cruel*, *horrid*, and even *li-li*. Some names would not be appropriate for me to mention here, and for those names we just shortened them down to the first letters; for example, *l b* meant "little b."

Can you name yours?

Importantly, this is also where a professional should come in to help. At first, your odap will *not* like it that you are getting honest with yourself *and* letting someone else in to help you. In its eyes, you do *not* need anyone else, and listening to *it* (the bestial character camouflaged via a rhetorical voice) is the best choice you can and will ever make, if you want to lose weight, that is!

In using these rhetorical strategies, this gremlin—or if you wish, devilish addiction personality—incarcerates the potential processed food addict through its ever so well-known voice. This is where its power and control originate. What is so devilish about this part of the disease of processed food addiction—a part that is rarely, if ever, spoken about—is the means by which it takes over. It likes to stay invisible, which is why it remains so deceptive, probing the potential addict and saying *they* are the problem.

Over time, it uses this invisible, reiterating, bestial voice to convince the individual that they are "the fat one, the overweight one, the mentally unstable one ..."

The odap's cunning nature is so convincing that the person believes the problem actually emanates from themselves, forming an unambiguous line between the person and the problem. In other words, they think, "I must be the one with the deranged mind," which keeps the odap in disguise. No wonder medical professionals, family, friends, and colleagues do not have a clue what is really going on. As a result, when talking to the addict, even the professionals usually base their questions on the assumption that the addict is the disorder.

Jennifer Shares

> I knew something was wrong with me but I did not know what. I just couldn't stop ingesting processed foods like my friends seemed to be able to do. I tried all types of things, until one day I became suicidal. I knew something was wrong, but I couldn't place what it was, and I thought it was much easier to die than to go on living and facing this every day.

> I was placed in an anorexic-bulimic clinic, but later down the track, after an actual suicide attempt, I was placed in a psych ward and diagnosed with schizophrenia and given the appropriate meds. I and all the professional and non-professional people around me were trying to fix me. My disease of addiction was buried once again.

> I do not want to say anyone was at fault here, as all of us involved were none the wiser.

> I knew there was something wrong with me. So all I needed was some new thinking—thoughts that could replace the ones that were relentlessly going on and new ones to help me to learn how to control my crazy thoughts. Those crazy thoughts always seemed at the end of the day to come back to my junk food intake, or my weight, or how I looked, or how pathetic, hopeless, unworthy I was.

> I have since learned that it was the processed food I was ingesting that made me crazy. I needed to somehow obtain an inactive processed food addiction personality.

> Thankfully, I have had effective treatment and my disease of PFA is in remission.

However, a word of warning: I am very cautious of the fact that I am just one bite away from a binge. I know that one crumb of processed food in any form (even overeating on non-processed food can spark off my craving) can reactivate my quiescent personality, returning me to the merciless insanity of processed food addiction.

Even more disturbing and disheartening is the fact that, externally, processed food addicts look relatively normal. No one can really know or understand the torture, the relentless torment, the fears, and the anxiety they endure throughout the day. No other method of torture, whether traditional, corporal, or alternative punishment, is needed for the disease to keep destroying the potential processed food addict's body, mind, and spirit.

Over the years, I have had some patients do drawings of their disease voice, resulting in some interesting works of art. I am often amazed by how this is another step in breaking the denial of what is actually happening for the individual. A large part of helping a processed food addict to recover is gaining their trust, which the devilish addict personality (gremlin) ultimately tries to destroy in its victims.

Every time a person (professional or not) attempts to get close enough to understand what is happening for the processed food addict, the bestial gremlin flips whatever the person is saying and boomerangs it back so that it's always the addict's fault. As this disease progresses, the addict will usually lose trust in those around them, in society, and ultimately in themselves.

As they say, addiction is an obsession of the mind, and this is where it begins. Once again, this illness is a disease of denial—denial of the mind. "One day I will be able to control and enjoy my processed food intake."

The processed food addict thinks the solution to all of her problems is just to lose weight. This remedy, according to odap, is for anyone and everyone, whether overweight, healthy weight, or underweight. In fact, I have seen people who may have early to mid-stage processed food addictions but were able to stop and eliminate processed food for a considerable amount of time. The problem here is that the person believes if she stays *empty* now, she will be able to control and enjoy her processed food when she gets older and will be able to enjoy her grandkids.

Nelly Shares

> *I stopped eating processed foods several decades ago (in my late thirties), as they were hindering me being able to be a good mother to my kids. I didn't travel to all those places I dreamed of visiting, but instead saved up my money to share with my children and their families when I retired.*
>
> *With this in mind and through self-discipline, willpower, and control, which I had exhibited over the past thirty years, when I finally got my longed-for grandkids, I was sure that I could now ingest processed foods like other people.*
>
> *So, I booked us all on a two-week cruise—me, my family, and their children (my grandkids). However, within six months, I had put back on all the weight plus some that I had kept off for over thirty years.*
>
> *Once again, I tried to eliminate the processed foods just like I had done when I was in my thirties. However, the more methods I tried to control the processed foods—and even new ones that were now available, which I could afford easily—I found it was impossible for me to do so!!!*

This reiterates the maxim "Once a processed food addict, always a processed food addict." Starting to ingest processed foods after any length of time abstaining leads to being off again, only worse than before. Processed food addicts have binged from being full of guilt, depression, anxiety, and despair, or alternatively, binged to celebrate feeling happy, successful, elated, and excited. It does not matter what the feelings and thoughts are when a bio-psycho-social-spiritual phenomenon is at play and the negative voice is active: its ulterior motive is for the processed food addict to eat in a manner that brings on psychosis or death, while mouthing one of its never-ending mantras, "This time it will be different," "One won't hurt you," "You have been so good, so why not?," or "You're at your goal weight now, showing you can finally control it."

This denial continues to grow, but so does the disease in so many ways. The processed food addict's secret (most often subliminal) pessimistic gremlin (odap) is perpetually opposing the person's Jiminy Cricket voice (the person's conscience, inner spirit, or sixth sense). These two voices are constantly playing out in the mind of a processed food addict and are so delusional that the processed food addict cannot, after a time, discern reality from deception. This keeps alive the mental obsession that they will be able to beat it and that somehow they are different from other people who succumbed to the illness. This negative mentality progresses to become the dominant force in the processed food addict's mind.

It is essential for me to state this at the beginning of treatment for someone with a processed food addiction. A processed food addict typically believes that she and this voice are one and the same entity. In recovery, it is important that I separate the person from the voice that delineates circumstances, making potential addicts vulnerable to the mental obsession that rhetorically seduces a person into believing promises—promises that are in fact illusional (unreal visions) and delusional (false beliefs), which they are powerless over.

Naomi Shares

> *What a relief to learn that all I am is a processed food addict, and more important for me was not only learning this truth BUT understanding "It was NOT my fault!" I was not to blame and those feelings of guilt, remorse, fear, and self-pity that systemically infiltrated my whole being were only different guises of the disease.*

You see, from as far back as I can remember, "dh" (which stood for d_ _ _head) was a part of my thinking. It made infinite sweet promises to end my physical and mental suffering, AND it pledged to make my dreams and hopes a reality. Dh would tell me over and over again how worthless I was, that I wouldn't amount to anything, that I would always be as big as a house, and that I would never get or sustain a job.

It would say, "People like you aren't worthy of anything because you're so fat and lazy," and then it would do this twist in my thinking. My addictionologist calls it "the flip."

Dh would then flip around and even call me by name, which made me believe in its rhetorical voice even more, Argh!

"BUT perhaps, Naomi, there may be some hope for you. You may even be able to change, and in the process, I will help you be more in control, more loveable, more worthy, and even more perfect. BUT in order to do this, you will have to trust no one but me, do what I say without question, as I am the only one that understands you. Don't you remember? I have always looked out for you and had your best interests at heart. The answer is actually quite simple, BUT it will be hard for someone like you to accomplish. BUT if you commit to me, stay in control, use your willpower, and work like your life depends on it (which I need to remind you it does), then I believe you can and WILL do it. What is the answer? That is simple. Do whatever you have to do to lose weight."

How I loved this empty promise! This answer seemed to be inked on my soul; my whole life revolved around it. I wanted nothing more in this world than to lose weight. I have since talked with other recovered processed food addicts who were a healthy weight but it convinced them that they looked like the Michelin Man.

How I believed these promises, day in and day out, for far too long. Dh gave me the illusion that I could fix it. That I was the problem BUT I was fixable.

I only had to look around me and see so many other girls and women who were normal weight or even a little bit heavier BUT they could control AND enjoy how much pizza and garlic bread they ate. Even have some dessert and stop.

Needless to say, the fingers then always pointed back at me. And of course, me being a perfectionist, I had to always do what was expected of me. So I was the problem once again.

Even professionals spoke to me as if I was the problem. I had this psychiatric disorder coupled with emotional instability. So I found myself playing the game—yep, I'm the problem, all right. Anything for me to say and do in order to fix this thing. I was all in!

In recovery today, I've learned that it doesn't matter what I do. I will never be able to ingest processed foods like normal people. Just like someone with diabetes will never be able to fix their pancreas. I now can spot dh's voice straight up and turn toward my own little voice, which continues to become louder and louder as my disease of processed food addiction stays in remission.

I am discovering me—who I am, my desires, my goals, my dreams, what are my career choices. The devilish addict personality has dissipated so much.

I now can see that when I was at my most vulnerable (sick and desperate), this disease was about 85 percent (plus or minus) dictating my life, and I was lucky to have 20 percent (plus or minus) on a good day.

Over time, it is easy to spot the driven rhetorical voice automatically taking over the person's thinking—"One won't hurt you"—even against their own will. With this display of deception, the processed food addict has no resistance against ingesting that first bite of processed food. Conversely, at times, the processed food addict willingly complies with the voice out of fear, elation, guilt, and the like, even blaming themselves, totally unaware they have a bio-psycho-social-spiritual disease dictating their thoughts, behavior, and personality.

Even though the disease begins in the mind, it is bio-psycho-social-spiritual, not just mental. Thus, all areas of addiction must be treated if the processed food addict is to experience longevity in recovery with peace of mind from this malady.

Sometimes, potential processed food addicts will open up and share with a clinician some minimal semblance of what is going on: the pain, torture, and fears. It is quite rare for them to open up—and is dependent on what stage the addiction has taken them to—and then walk out with a mental health diagnosis. The treatment has been to fix or at least hinder the thoughts, which is similar to treating depression. This all sounds good and may be a valid panacea for those not suffering from a disease of addiction; however, unless the primary illness is dealt with first (i.e., the addiction), the secondary symptoms will continue. This brings me again to reiterate the point of how important it is for the professional to have specialized education and training in the diagnosis and treatment of the disease of addiction.

With each day that I treat processed food addiction, I wholeheartedly believe it is a unitary disorder. I agree that in the genesis of processed food addiction, both nature and nurture play important roles; however, critical investigations and research are yet to be accomplished.

Powerlessness

I would like to keep this piece on powerlessness simple. Hence, following on from the physical and mental elements of the disease of processed food addiction, we will now visit this notion of powerlessness that is bandied around.

The mind of a processed food addict is out to destroy the body, and yet the body is destroying the mind (through physical craving).

A processed food addict cannot ingest processed foods because of the body (the physical craving to want more), and they cannot quit because of the obsession of the mind (trying with all their willpower to somehow, one day, be able to ingest processed foods like *normal* people). This is coupled with a strong rhetorical voice ("It's okay, just one bite won't hurt you—it will be different this time").

What's more, this phenomenon of craving is limited to addicts only and never occurs in the majority of people. This being so, the processed food addict is powerless over their inability to control and enjoy their ingestion of processed foods; and then, of course, their life becomes unmanageable in trying to accomplish such a task. This makes an addict powerless over their addictive substance, which in turn makes for an unmanageable life—the mind and body self-destructing each other.

A Spiritual Solution

A spiritual solution is a psychic change brought about primarily by the addict understanding the disease of addiction, eliminating the cause (that is, all processed food), and then being able to think more clearly and learn how to treat their disease. With a spiritual solution, a person becomes more and more honest with themselves each day, as recovery is spiritually centered.

There is a lot of literature nowadays about spirituality, different religions, and the holistic journeys individuals take. I tend to see the spiritual element as basically regarding a person's usefulness and purpose in life. This provides a spiritual equilibrium for the basic instincts of human nature: (1) society, meaning relationships with friends, family, and the world around us; (2) security, meaning monetary status and emotional security; and (3) sexual activity, meaning innate desires for an acceptable sex life. Simply stated, a spiritual solution is getting honest with oneself.

Typically, addiction is a disease of denial (once again, denial). And the most life-preserving quality of honesty for any person suffering from processed food addiction is understanding and accepting the fact that they have this illness known as addiction and there is nothing they can do about this fact, other than treat it. This is ego-deflation at its best—humility. This humility is found by facing the fact that processed food addiction is a fatal malady over which the addict is individually powerless to change.

The good news is that it can go into remission one day at a time, and the processed food addict can live a happy and holistic life, better than before when they had a full-blown addiction. The billion-dollar question is: Are you willing to eliminate the substance and adopt a new way of living?

Nora Shares

Nora came into my clinic wanting an answer to "fix this thing." She complained how sad it was at home, that her daughter and son saw her ingest processed foods daily and were disgusted by how much weight she put on. They bore witness innumerable times to Nora's promises that this diet would be the diet to end all diets.

Nora shared how bad she felt and that her husband had paid so much money over the years to fix her. She felt so sorry for him, having to look after her and continually keep paying for her latest adventure in proving she could do this all by herself.

She shared, "Poor Henry, my husband. I feel so bad for him, as he just tries so hard to help me. I am worried about all the money he has spent to help me ..."

I stopped her mid-sentence and said, "Nora, it is a simple answer. Ask for help *and stop* ingesting the processed foods. Put the lid on the cookie jar, and then Henry won't have to keep forking out all this money. I will pull you all the way, but I won't push you. Your desire to get well must come from you, from within."

Surprisingly (*not* surprising, in fact), Nora would do anything *but* stop ingesting processed foods. She still thought she could fix it herself. This is where the ego-deflation comes in. In life there are some things we cannot control; although if you are a potential processed food addict, I would assume your odap is saying something along the lines of "That is such bull! I'll show her."

I often say to patients in the preliminary days of treatment, "There is a red door, a yellow door, and a green door. You can go in and out of the red door and the green door, but you cannot go through the yellow door. Which door do you want to go through the most?"

More often than not, it will be the yellow door, especially if they are a severe processed food addict. This writing is not about the personality makeup of a processed food addict, nor is it about classifying them into specific categories—that would be an almost impossible task. However, what I do believe and stand by unconditionally is that severe processed food addicts have the primary manifestation of the disease of addiction in common—once they ingest processed food, the phenomenon of craving will develop, and this is what makes them different from other folks. In my experience this malady has never been cured, as with other non-communicable diseases.

An addict will do anything but willingly surrender the substance unless they have had enough or have an honest desire to get well. They can play the game and say how sorry they are about this and that and how awful it is, but they won't eliminate the substance unless they have to do so to stay alive themselves. This conversation can be quite typical for a processed food addict; they will do anything *but* eliminate the processed foods. You see, processed foods were not Nora's problem: it was learning to function without them—this was the core of the problem.

Hence the solution for treating the disease of addiction (getting honest with oneself and holistically learning how to implement a new life without ingesting processed foods) seems like a tall order to the majority of those inflicted with this malady.

Observational evidence continues to show that a processed food addict may be genetically predisposed to the disease of addiction. There are several different programs and eating plans, all aiming to eliminate the problem foods. This is but a mere beginning to treating the disease of processed food addiction, as treating the addiction in this way is only really touching the surface of the problem; only the substance has been eliminated.

As shown by Nora's story, it is not living with the processed foods that is the problem, it is learning *how to live without them*. If one just goes on an elimination diet or food plan, then that is all that is done. The processed food addict usually ends up as an "empty processed food addict," who sooner or later has a huge relapse. The bust may start off with just a little bit here and there, as nothing has changed. The person is trying to fix the problem *with* the problem, doing all they can to control their ingestion of processed foods (fix the problem) with one thought in mind: "I have to lose weight or I am not worthy of living."

Foremost in the recovery of a person shown to have high symptomology of processed food addiction, it is essential to eliminate the substance—all processed foods. This is known as *abstinence*. Abstaining from processed foods includes eliminating all processed and refined foods and high-fat foods, and abstaining from *volumizing*, which is overeating non-processed foods.

Once the processed food addict becomes abstinent, the question is, how do they stay abstinent with peace of mind, especially when they have tried all the avenues known to mankind to not ingest processed foods. Moreover, they are abetted in this blindness by a society that does not comprehend the difference between sane eating and processed food addiction.

The first stage of recovery from processed food addiction is finding out if one is a processed food addict or not, followed immediately by professional information from an addiction specialist as to what to do about it. Education involves the processed food addict surrounding themselves with recovered people and attending support groups to nullify the disease's ammunition—**isolation**. In turn, the addict will cultivate honesty, open-mindedness, and willingness to consult with an addictionologist or specialist in the treatment of their addiction, if deemed necessary for complete recovery.

Let's simplify some key points I have been working toward regarding the "threefold disease" concept of addiction, since it appears to baffle so many. When treating addiction, I often need to explain things in different ways for the processed food addict to gain a greater understanding of this malady.

When recovery is sought for processed food addiction, generally it will be primarily on the physical plane, so to speak, that is, involving the physical symptoms (obesity, being underweight, diet-binge cycles, purging, laxative abuse, gall bladder issues, irregular menstrual cycles, and mouth and gum disease, just to name a few). The concentration is on losing weight. However, even when weight loss does occur (if we don't drink, we won't get drunk; if we don't ingest processed foods, we won't get fat), the weight, which is in reality only a symptom of the disease, will pile back on again. Efforts are then increased to try to control it further.

Then the processed food addict decides that since that didn't work, "this thing" must be psychological. So they sign up for weight-loss surgery options to motivate themselves to lose the weight pre-op; enroll in the latest CBT, ACT, and mindfulness courses; or attend health retreats and food addiction workshops. All this is an attempt to fix the emotions and prevent relapses, plus gain some control back, and while doing so, start the latest diet, food plan, or other method of control. They believe while they are fixing their emotions and their unmanageable life, there will be no need to binge (ingest processed foods). *But* after several weeks or perhaps even months (depending on the control method), the mental twist takes over again. They may take a bite without even thinking about it, or plan the binge feeling justified by anger, fear, worry, or jealousy. Whatever their reason, given the usual consequences of a binge, their justification for a spree is utterly senseless.

Then they hear the word *spiritual* and think it must mean "join a religion." Many do join different religious bodies, even going to the point of being confirmed. One patient became a monk to seek God so he would not ingest processed food or alcohol, which were destroying his soul. But this search still led him back to the processed foods eventually.

Dr. Robert Smith, who is known as the co-founder of Alcoholics Anonymous, in his farewell speech, emphasized the point of keeping it simple:

> *There are two or three things that flashed into my mind on which it would be fitting to lay a little emphasis. One is the simplicity of our program. Let's not louse it all up with Freudian complexes and things that are interesting to the scientific mind but have very little to do with our actual AA work. Our Twelve Steps, when simmered down to the last, resolve themselves into the words "love" and "service." We understand what love is, and we understand what service is. So, let's bear those two things in mind. Let us also remember to guard that erring member, the tongue, and if we must use it, let's use it with kindness and consideration and tolerance.*[11]

In treating people who have an addiction diagnosis, I continue to find that "keeping it simple" plays an integral role in the methodology of ensuring the disease stays in remission—that is, the person experiencing permanent abstinence and sobriety, *with peace of mind*, one day at a time. Working on the mind of an addict with Freudian approaches (psychoanalysis) only feeds the disease of denial.

How? you may ask. While the addict is working on their psychological behaviors, dysfunctional relationships, compulsivity, or the manifestations of a negligent upbringing, they are able to continue to deny that they are a real addict, that they have a bio-psycho-social-spiritual thing, a whole-life thing, happening. Once a processed food addict, always a processed food addict.

Science may one day change this, but it hasn't done so yet, for processed food addiction or any other addiction. Yes, it is true the

---

[11] Alcoholics Anonymous World Services, Inc., 1980, p. 338

aggregate number of people who recover using psychiatric methods is appreciable; however, there appear to be quite a few individuals who have not experienced sustained recovery with peace of mind via psychological, psychiatric, or surgical methods.

Once again (repetition is the mother of wisdom), spirituality is about being honest with yourself: "to thine own self be true." This is easier said than done. Unfortunately, the pains of eating processed foods must come before abstinence, and the pains of emotional turmoil come before serenity.

Another lesson, one that I find very helpful in keeping this spiritual aspect simple, is coming to understand that there is a higher power (a higher being, a deity, God, a creator, a divine intelligence, Nature) and it is not *me*! Often someone suffering from a chronic illness will ask people to pray for them. If you have been diagnosed with the disease of processed food addiction, there is nothing you can do to change this diagnosis; all you can do is accept it and get it treated. I have found with patients that some are very much anti-God (atheists) and some don't care whether there might be a God or not, they just want to be left alone and do what they want to do when they want to do it, relying on their own intelligence and self-sufficiency (agnostics). Then there are, of course, some who believe wholeheartedly that "Yes, there is a God and He is everything" (theists). If or when this question arises, I like to say that what you believe in is no one else's business. The first footprint of recovery is to understand the disease of processed food addiction and all its ramifications. Furthermore, when you abstain from processed foods, your brain becomes clearer and that inner knowing (inner voice, intuition, sixth sense, ESP) is not blocked off from the inner voice. So, you can think more rationally and hear your inner voice, your sixth sense, or as I call it, your Jiminy Cricket, more clearly.

In summary, recovery has three fundamental features: getting treatment for the processed food addiction, being involved in a community that supports recovering from this malady, and developing a spiritual way of life to support and aid consistent and permanent recovery from this progressive disease, one day at a time.

Chapter Nine

Touching on Relapse

elapse has garnered a bad name for itself in treatment of the disease of addiction, which somehow paves the way for the notion that addicts are different from other human beings. I see in the clinic that there is nothing unpredictable about an addict relapsing, just as there is nothing unpredictable about a person with type 2 diabetes (t2d), cardiac disease, or cancer—or a chronic illness, for that matter—enduring a relapse. I believe addicts are the same as all other people. They are characteristic of all humanity, as are people with other chronic diseases.

I liken an addict relapsing (also known as a bust, a slip, a setback, a recurrence, a failed treatment) to be analogous with other people who experience a relapse. A person with t2d, hypertension, mental illnesses, or cardiovascular disease, for example, is prescribed a binding and vigorous treatment schedule. If the person breaches their treatment, they may experience very little effect in the short term. However, with a bit more time, as they start to ignore other instructions given by the treating clinician, then sooner or later, they experience a relapse. Most normal human beings decide they are the exception to the rule, different, and they don't have to follow the directions given. This seems to be an inherent part of human nature. Such is life! It is apparent everywhere, not just among processed food addicts, alcoholics, or addicts, but within society as a whole today.

More importantly, it is clear how relapse can be prevented. It is critical that the patient has a complete understanding of the nature of their disease (how it occurs, how it affects them in all aspects of their life—brain functioning, behaviors, thinking, personality—why they will relapse if they do not treat their disease, and why they cannot stop treating their condition without experiencing a relapse). In short, these fundamental questions must be confronted, answered, and reiterated while the patient learns to follow the directions of the treating clinician today, tomorrow, and post recovery.

I do not differentiate between people suffering from chronic conditions. I believe there is no more reason to speak of "the processed food addict mind" than to try to describe "the diabetic mind" or "the cardiac mind." I find in clinic that my effectiveness in treating addiction is greatly increased when I can help the patient recognize and understand that they are only human, afflicted with human nature.

What actions are in order to prevent a relapse?

The topic of the actions required to prevent a relapse is one that has been researched and written about in addiction literature for decades. A bust, a slip, or a relapse is a clear acknowledgement that regardless of all the knowledge you have gained and with the best efforts you could muster thus far to stay abstinent, you have picked up (ingested) processed foods again. What is important to understand is that with many chronic illnesses, such as diabetes mellitus, the disease may be under control and then suddenly the sufferer can have high blood glucose levels, meaning the disease has flared up again. This is also true for the disease of addiction. It is quite common for an addict to slip (especially in the first days and weeks of abstinence). Hence, it is important to understand the relapse process and, if it does happen, to put action in place so that it does not continue to occur.

Usually an individual relapses because she has skipped some of her meals, overexerted herself, decided to see if she could control her intake of processed foods now that she knows better, or decided she is not losing weight fast enough, so "I may need to take back control again."

I just want to reiterate once again, weight gain is a symptom—a consequence of processed food addiction—not the cause. If an addict treats their processed food addiction, the weight will dissipate and stabilize. This is similar to alcoholics; if they don't drink alcohol, they won't get drunk.

As I have said, there is a myriad of reasons why we pick up after a period of abstaining from processed foods. I have come to see the patterns of behavior and thinking that underlie quite a lot of cases of relapsing into ingesting processed foods, again! Primarily, the processed food addict's worthiness, body-image, and self-esteem have been shot to pieces. For years, negative self-talk has been telling them lies such as "You'll never be thin and you're way too unworthy to even try that new job," and "No one will want to work with you because you're too fat and lazy." I'm sure you can add your own lies in here. It is no wonder that the processed food addict's self-esteem is practically nonexistent. Even triggers like losing a job, not getting a job, failing a course, losing a game of chess, or not passing a driving test can all damage a super-sensitive processed food addict with very feeble self-esteem. Of course, this makes the addict feel worse than they already did, so their default mechanism is always steering their thoughts to cupcakes or ice cream, instantaneously.

Any feelings of unworthiness breed self-pity, which goes hand in hand with a negative outlook on life. Downstream from this is feeling depressed, and then the processed food addict will find they are asking themselves, "What's the use of trying to abstain? I felt better when I was eating processed foods than I do now." An *empty* processed food addict only comprehends one thought! The only way to make these horrendous feelings go away is to eat, eat, eat, which then reinforces the belief that this is what makes them feel better. *This is treating the problem with the problem.*

As the proverb goes, if you lie down with dogs, you get up with fleas. Likewise, if you continually stay in a practicing environment, with the same people, places, and things around which you used to ingest processed food, you will pick up. This could be as simple as calling into a coffee shop or stopping by the 7-Eleven or the bakery where you used to get your food stash. Or it could be going where you used to go most often when you binged; staying in close contact with your eating buddies; attending morning teas, dinners, parties, and social catch-up events where processed food is served in abundance; keeping stashes of processed food around the house, just in case; hanging around the food courts of shopping centers; or walking past the takeouts you used to buy your supplies from. So, it is important to learn to not put yourself in an at-risk environment that may spark off the physical memories of processed food use and abuse, unless you have a valid reason to be at that particular place. We don't try to beat temptation, we avoid it!

Sometimes, a processed food addict will believe that they are not a real processed food addict and that they are surely the exception to this rule. So, after a period of abstinence, they go out and test the field again. That is, they go out for dinner and try to eat food that has been processed, just to see if they can now handle it, or hope that something has changed and they can miraculously now eat like other people. Again I reiterate, even at this late stage, summing up our time together while reading this book: once a processed food addict, always a processed food addict. After ingesting just a morsel of processed food, they are way back to where they started in the first place, or even worse.

Other triggers can be sickness, pain, or not being able to handle success or failure.

A relapse-prevention session provides a good opportunity to reiterate the disease concept of processed food addiction and what it means, and to get down to the core of the disease. During the session, it is reiterated that the patient is a processed food addict and this will never change. Additionally, going over the events that led to the bust can bring them into a positive perspective. This can be seen as an opportunity to reiterate the disease concept of addiction, which is similar to other chronic diseases; that is, processed food addiction is treated on a daily basis. If a diabetic misses their insulin, they are headed for trouble. If a processed food addict ingests a crumb of processed food, sooner or later it will spark off the allergy and they will spiral into a well-known binge. Only the processed food addict can take responsibility for the treatment of their disease and become aware of the people, places, and things that could lead to a bust. Hence, implementing preventative measures, one day at a time, is critical to ensure this does not come into fruition now that they are in recovery from the disease of processed food addiction.

Let's Wind Up This Portion for Now

Once the addict is able to understand their condition, only then can they learn how to live with it. Of course, this is more challenging than just reading these words, as each potential processed food addict generally comes with a lot of baggage—estranged marriages, working life in chaos, dysfunctional family environments, and strained friendships. However, through effective treatment, it is possible to help the addict sort through the chaos and commence the repair job necessary for building a new life free of the addictive substance(s).

I find that when the processed food addict admits *and* accepts the fact that they are an addict (depending on the substance) and, just as importantly, commits to and abides by the daily directions as though their life depends on it (which it does—addiction is a chronic fatal disease), they then set up a foundation for recovery. This is critical in protecting themselves not only against their own physical and mental chemistry but also against the social pressures to ingest processed food, long after they have finished treatment. It is essential that the processed food addict learn this new way of life that will protect their abstinence and sobriety. Permanent recovery from the disease of addiction is possible, if the person honestly wants to get well *and* is willing to make the effort.

I like to say, the effectiveness of the treatment I present and work with for processed food addiction is measured by my doing myself out of a job. When a person addresses their addiction, learns how to treat it themselves, and is able to function in society without the substance, one day at a time, then I blessedly am doing myself out of a job—something I can rejoice in, while waiting to help free my next potential processed food addict from the slavery of processed food addiction. Together, we can!

CHAPTER TEN

Recovery Begins

What does it mean to recover from processed food addiction?

I hope by now you have begun to understand the various stages in the progression of processed food addiction, which are similar to those of other addictions. I would like to reiterate that not everyone is a processed food addict.

Let's have a look at alcoholism, as there are so many similarities between it and processed food addiction. Alcoholism was recognized as a problem centuries ago, with religious, social, and political associations forming to take a stance on the use, misuse, and effects of alcohol (Vaillant, 1995). The early temperance movements (1800s) primarily aimed to push individuals to temper their drinking, that is, to drink less alcohol. Some temperance movements concentrated on advising individuals to cut back or curb their overindulgence of hard spirits rather than urging 100-percent abstinence from alcohol. They also concentrated on moral reform rather than legal measures against alcohol. However, by the 1820s, the temperance movement began to promote a total abstinence philosophy—that is, total elimination of all alcohol.

In later years (1830s and 1840s), there were over five thousand temperance movements; for example, the Washington Temperance

Society was formed in April 1840 and several years later had an alleged membership of well over 600,000 members (numbers vary depending on the source). The only requirement for membership was personal abstinence from all intoxicating drinks; reports suggest only approximately 100,000 were reformed "drunkards"—the term *alcoholic* had not been created yet (Bliss, 1835).

Part of the effectiveness and success of the Alcoholics Anonymous movement can be attributed to the lessons learned from the former temperance and intemperance societies—in particular, the Washingtonians—as well as the Oxford Group, a Christian group founded in 1919 by Frank Buchman, a Lutheran minister.[12] The Oxford Group's tenets became the bedrock for several notions in recovery from alcoholism (Wilson, 1957).

Similar to our predecessors in alcohol reform, movements have been and continue to be formed to address the trends of being overweight and having disordered eating. Primarily, the hazards of these trends and the many secondary complications resulting from overingesting processed foods have bred a myriad of diets, weight-loss schemes, and control methods over the centuries to combat the continual dramatic increase in the rates of obesity. On the other hand, social movements such as the fat-acceptance movement have emerged to change the anti-fat biases in societal attitudes.[13]

The first self-help group for overeating based on AA's 12 step program, Overeaters Anonymous (OA), came in the 1960s and offered an alternative approach to conventional dieting methods. Abstinence was defined as abstaining from compulsive overeating by implementing an eating plan. The original food plan was the "Gold Sheet" (later known as the "Grey Sheet Diet"), consisting of no refined carbohydrates. Through the years, the original OA group splintered into alternative self-help groups, all offering members different plans of

---

[12] Bill W., 1944
[13] Puhl & Heuer, 2010

abstinence.[14] The food plan of Food Addicts Anonymous advocates for all members to abstain from eating sugar, flour, and wheat products (1995). The main commonality among the 12 step food programs is a plan of eating, with slight variations in the food plan across programs, plus a 12 step way of life.

Coming forward to the twenty-first century, it continues to become clearer that it is near impossible for a *minority* of people to adhere to a food plan controlling how much they ingest, or to abstain from ingesting processed foods or particularly troublesome foods with peace of mind. Self-knowledge avails a processed food addict nothing. Once again, this is similar to alcoholism. For a *minority* of people who drink alcohol, they too are unable to control or stop their alcohol consumption on a continuing basis. As they strive to hold on to promises of serenity, peace, freedom from fear, and the like, which others appear to experience to varying degrees, they attempt to "do it again" and again, and again—get back on the food plan, get back on the wagon, hoping against hope that this time they will get it. While this is taking place, the "itty-bitty shitty committee" (odap) gets noisier and louder.

The point I am making is that nothing, to my knowledge, has been established to address processed food addiction for that minority of individuals who are 100 percent powerless, similar to the "drunkards" in the nineteenth and twentieth centuries who could not maintain a sober state with peace of mind. They always went back and drank again.

This book is founded on this fact. I treat persons who have crossed the so-called physiological line into addiction—from which there is no return, other than entire abstinence from processed foods. This is coupled with a continual understanding and acceptance of the disease concept of addiction, while implementing a spiritual way of life.

I encourage those I treat for addiction to attend the 12 step support groups of PFA, AA, NA, and Al-Anon. My work is to treat the disease

---

[14] Goldberg, 2003

of addiction—working with the addict to help them understand the nature of their disease, including understanding how it occurs; how it has affected their brains, their characters, and their actions; why processed foods must be avoided at all costs, every day; why they cannot safely ingest processed foods without sparking off the phenomenon of craving; and most importantly, why they will return to ingesting processed foods if their disease is not treated.

I am establishing a foundation for a new way of life, one that does not include ingesting processed food. I find that as the processed food addict surrenders to the fact that PFA is an irreversible disease and commits themselves to doing whatever it takes to keep the disease in remission, then, over time, their acceptance grows. This is a disease and there is nothing they can do to make themselves a normal eater, just as there is nothing a person with diabetes can do to think down their blood sugar or a person with cardiac disease can do to run a marathon.

Although in treating the disease of processed food addiction I strive for permanent abstinence and a contented, useful life (akin to AA), part of the surrender and acceptance process is relapse—two steps forward, one step back.[15] Addiction is a deadly disease, and like all diseases, it too comes with relapses. For example, a person with diabetes may be traveling along with their blood sugar levels balanced, and then they may miss their insulin intake, or indulge in a lot of junk food, or let up on their daily exercise regime, and find themselves in a distressing hypoglycemic state. Once again, their disease has come to the fore, reminding them that they have diabetes and it has to be treated on a daily basis. Over time, it becomes much easier to treat their disease each day than to go through the relapse again—paving the way for the acceptance of having a disease, knowing it is treatable, and accepting that there is nothing they can do to change it.

A person is either pregnant or they are not; one cannot be half pregnant.

---

[15] *Twelve Steps and Twelve Traditions*, 1988, p. 40

The notion that the processed food addict is similar to other people or that at present they are able to control and enjoy ingesting processed foods has to be annihilated.

Unfortunately, I have witnessed competition in the arena of recovery from disordered eating, both in weight-loss groups and support groups. The competition resides in whoever has lost the most weight or been abstinent the longest, seems to somehow be the expert, is doing that particular program perfectly, or has some special connection to God. There is *no* competition if someone's cancer has been in remission for five years and someone else's cancer has been in remission for five months. More likely, there is love, support, compassion, hope, and joy in escaping from a chronic and sometimes fatal malady.

I say, "The person who woke up the earliest this morning and treated their disease throughout the day has been the longest in recovery today."

> The person who woke up the earliest this morning and treated their disease throughout the day has been the longest in recovery today.
>
> The Author

So, whether one does or does not relapse in the early stages of recovery is not the matter to address. For me, the question is, What can I do to help the potential addict to further understand that this is a disease? AA's *Twelve Steps and Twelve Traditions* states, "Pain is the touchstone of all spiritual progress" (1988, p. 93). In recovering from processed food addiction, the pains of ingesting processed foods had to come before understanding and abstinence, and the pains of emotional turmoil before peace of mind and serenity.

Is what I have written thus far inapplicable to the majority of society? The answer is, definitely not. You may not have crossed the physiological line to being a real processed food addict, but you could be in the earlier stages of processed food abuse. Just like in the temperance movements of the past, whose members actually found a way of living while tempering their alcohol consumption, so too can anyone take steps to prevent progressing to the later stages of addiction, once they are privy to the knowledge of what processed food addiction is.

So, stated simply, not everyone is a real processed food addict! Yes, there are many and varied persons diagnosed with eating disorders, food misuse, food abuse, compulsive overeating, binge eating disorder (BED), bulimia, anorexia, and more. And more importantly, they are being treated accordingly. However, in today's society we have what's termed a *real processed food addict*. This is akin to the *real alcoholics* of the past, who *could not temper* their alcohol consumption. As much as they would have liked to, it was impossible.

Even high functioning addicts (HFA)—who may be extremely overweight, or underweight and vomiting their last binge down the toilet—may be getting away with denial for now. But sooner or later, the disease will progress to blotting out their unbearable situation as best they can, or finally facing up to reality and asking for help, not because they have to but because they want to and are willing to exert themselves to do whatever it takes to get well and stay well.

I have witnessed individuals with health complications—including obesity, type 2 diabetes, prediabetes, cardiac disease, cancer, severe chronic migraines, and disordered eating—who have made an informed decision to *temper* their processed food intake. They came to understand that processed foods may be a significant part of their physical and mental dysfunctionality, so tempering their processed food ingestion paid dividends in all areas of their life.

Conversely, I have also treated processed food addicts who presented with a type 2 diabetes diagnosis, were on medications for their diabetes, and were in psychological distress (depression, anxiety, and stress) and who, try as they might, could not stick to any low glycemic diet consistently. Sooner or later, the mental twist would kick in and they would find themselves with their heads in the cookie jar, berating themselves for "doing it again." Their diabetes management plan went out the window.

After treatment for the disease of processed food addiction, they were given a blood test, called an A1c, that showed their average levels of blood glucose over the past three months. They were able to achieve A1c levels between 4 and 5.6 percent, not by following a very strict diabetes management and diet regimen (which is impossible if one is a processed food addict), but through the recognition of a processed food addiction diagnosis. They treated the cause—processed food addiction—and the secondary complications dissipated.

Primarily, treatment begins by eliminating the processed foods, followed closely by helping the patient to understand what an addiction is. We address topics like the "Why me?" syndrome, the hidden stages of addiction, psychological influences and consequences, and why it was necessary to continually ingest more and more processed foods to function as the disease progressed (tolerance and withdrawal symptomology). A person cannot continue to implement change if they do not know *and understand* why, and what the problem is, and why it is imperative that the changes take place.

Ultimately, though, it is up to the patient. If someone still wants to do it their way—that is, fight reality via denial and try to control their processed food consumption themselves—then that is their choice. Ultimately, if one is a processed food addict, the disease will progress; it will only get worse, never better. Sometimes individuals have to go back out and try the old game again, until they have had enough and want to change. The desire for long-term, permanent recovery, one day at a time, must come from within. Of course, this is a very brief description of treating the disease of processed food addiction.

I will endeavor to go into more depth on the process of treating processed food addiction at another time in the near future.

I also find in addiction treatment and recovery that a large part of what I do is to not enable the potential processed food addict. It is important they start to be responsible for their choices, their actions, and their behaviors. Yes, they are powerless over the diagnosis of being a processed food addict, but they are not powerless over asking and seeking help to change and treat their disease. The message I would like to pass on to our health professionals, families, friends, neighbors, and colleagues is this: processed food addiction is a disease separate from disordered eating; it is treatable and it can go into remission.

As I and others continue to emphasize that processed food addiction is an illness, the social stigma associated with this condition will dissipate, and hopefully one day historians will recognize processed food addiction in its entirety—a disease similar to other substance-use disorders. I hope we can all unite and, even though an individual may not be a real (severe) processed food addict, be proactive in helping them take steps toward protecting themselves from secondary complication as they age.

What are processed foods?

As I say in chapter 1, this is a really important question. A good place to start is to ask yourself, "What are highly refined, processed foods, and what are junk foods?" As previously stated, if one is an alcoholic, abstinence necessitates abstaining from all alcoholic beverages, drinking only tea, coffee, orange juice, milk, water, and the like. Similarly, the processed food addict abstains from all processed foods, ingesting only lean protein, fruit, vegetables, salads, carbohydrates (whole grains and complex starches), oil (unsaturated fats, including polyunsaturated fatty acids and monounsaturated fats) and low-fat dairy products (<0.01% fat).

Yes, some argue that most foods, whether natural, organic, or whatever, have been tampered with in some way, shape, or form. But let's say, for example, that a processed food addict drinks skim milk and eats non-fat plain yogurt (<0.01% fat). Yes, it has gone through the manufacturing stages; however, because it has almost no artificial sugars or high fats, it does not trigger the phenomenon of craving. There is a similar scenario with fats. Olive oil and healthier fats (monounsaturated *and* polyunsaturated) do not hijack the brain like saturated *and* trans fats do in some people. Additionally, if a processed food addict ingests too much of any non-processed foods, it will eventually lead them back to ingesting processed foods, as the processed food addict's brain and body know the only way to relieve the restlessness, irritability, and discontent they may be experiencing is to ingest processed food, the ultimate elixir. They are chasing the ease and comfort that comes from ingesting just one crumb of processed food, which will immediately numb out reality.

We say, "One's too many and a hundred are not enough!"

I was reading some research recently that told of a patient in alcohol rehab who started ingesting the hand sanitizer from the restroom. That is not the normal way one would drink alcohol; however, the patient's brain was still getting its hit and did not necessarily have to drink alcohol in a normal fashion.

Notably, there continues to be an upsurge in synthetic drugs, those created using man-made chemicals, for example, ecstasy. In the food industry this has already been labeled *artificial* instead of *synthetic*. The term *artificial* typically refers to ingredients or foods created to imitate nature, for example, certain colorings or flavors. In the twenty-first century, it has become apparent that scientific changes will continue to occur in food production, similar to the increase in the manufacture of synthetic drugs globally. Only time will gauge what the outcomes will be as research, literature, and clinical trials guide future developments in this area.

Preliminary Elimination of Processed Foods

The prescription for treating processed food addiction is the preliminary elimination of processed foods. The first requirement for treating this disease is to eliminate the source of the trouble—processed foods. We primarily treat the cause (processed foods) and not the symptoms of weight, depression, anxiety, and distress. If an alcoholic does not drink alcohol, they do not get drunk; similarly, if a processed food addict does not ingest processed foods, they don't put on weight.

Treatment consists of a guide detailing a baseline eating regime to ensure one has enough nutrients in one's system to stave off physiological hunger. Diets and prepared meals delivered to one's door have helped a multitude of people over the years. Indeed, in the pioneering times of trying to find an answer as to why people who were overindulging in junk food could not stop compulsive overeating, the first food plan was established.

The baseline prescription below has been developed from working clinically with processed food addicts. It details the type and amount of non-processed food to be consumed (by weight) to eliminate processed foods in the preliminary treatment stage of processed food addiction. This is pertinent in developing a new way of living—a new lifestyle that promotes and sustains one's recovery on a daily basis. However, eliminating processed foods is just the tip of the iceberg; that is why a food plan alone will not work for a processed food addict.

Through clinic work, I have changed somewhat the food plans originally used in treating compulsive overeating, disordered eating, and food addiction. Rather than measuring by cups, I recommend weighing the amount of non-processed foods. I have had several of my patients use this method and the successful results speak for themselves.

Grace Shares

By weighing instead of measuring my non-processed food, I feel I am getting the exact amount of food my brain needs. When measuring in cups and the like, my disease had room to play with the amount. For example, I'd be tempted to heap the cup or stuff the cup. My disease would tell me, "It's still only one cup if it fits in there." Sooner or later, this would set my disease off, because now volume (extra food) was hijacking my brain. With weighing, I'm getting the exact right amount every single time. This keeps my brain chemistry in balance and my disease of processed food addiction in remission.

Jane Shares

I have been recovered from processed food addiction for over three years now. I used to take my scales, measuring cups, and spoons everywhere I went. It felt like such a hassle to do this and I felt stigmatized to have all these measuring utensils spread out wherever I was going to eat my meal.

Today, I go to a restaurant with my Joseph Joseph TriScale, place my plate on top of the scale, and start weighing only. For example, I place my plate on the scale and measure 4 ounces of protein, add 10 ounces of cooked vegetables, and then add 6 ounces of rice!!! or 8 ounces of cooked potato. I then remove my plate, fold up the scales, put them back into my bag, and enjoy my meal without having measuring cups and utensils spread all over the table.

Most important for me is the freedom I now feel when I go out with my many business colleagues for lunch or dinner. No one says anything these days, and if they do, I just share I have an allergy to processed foods and this is what I do to stay abstinent. More often than not, I get positive feedback wishing they too could be as healthy as me.

Christine Shares

I live in Australia and I was reluctant to eat out due to the fact that people looked and stared when I got out all my weighing and measuring utensils at restaurants. I have found since that just using my scales not only enables me to eat my weighed meal without feeling different but I don't volumize or stuff my cup with extra food. I place my plate on top of my scales, measure out my meal quantity (protein, carbohydrate, and starch) and off I go.

People don't even look twice.

I treat my disease with the medicine (non-processed food) that I need and eat an abstinent meal (medicine) with peace of mind and no one looks twice. My brain and body are getting the right amount of fuel that I need, with no extra kicks from having a little

> *extra food ... extra food that always led me to the only elixir I knew. Weighing my food not only makes my life easier but it's also more convenient, as I just weigh and go.*
>
> *I also learned early on in my recovery that if the focus is still on the symptoms of my disease (weight, food, and so on) and not on the solution (elimination and taking the steps necessary to treat my disease daily), then I was still in the problem. Today, I focus on the solution, treating my disease of processed food addiction. I AM happy, joyous, and free today.*

The reason this change has occurred is that over time I found that quite a few processed food addicts had made a great start at recovery—that is, they had eliminated processed foods—but as their recovery continued and they started to learn how to face life instead of ingesting processed food to cope, the old symptoms of restlessness, irritability, and distress begin to prowl around. The processed food addict has come to understand and accept that it is fatal to ingest processed foods, so they start to stuff their cups with extra salad or vegetables, mound their cups of yogurt, lick spoons, and so on, justifying to themselves, "Well, at least it's non-processed food."

The most common justification for processed food addicts is when they get into dried fruit and nuts, believing and telling themselves, "They can't hurt me." This may not seem like a big deal to normal eaters, but for processed food addicts, it can and does lead them back to ingesting the only elixir they know—processed foods. At first, they see it as harmless, so they then add some extra food in other areas. Then they think, "That experiment went well, so perhaps I can now try some extra yogurt or dressing, or add some ketchup to my steamed potato, plus some coconut water or diet soda." That experiment goes well, so now they try some low-fat fruit yogurt. Sooner or later, they are trying some bakery items, while still rationalizing to themselves that "this time it will be different."

Once a processed food addict, always a processed food addict!

Another common aspect of the disease of addiction among those in recovery is the notion that because the urge to ingest, drink, and use is gone, they are cured or can now control it. This thinking has many an addict pick up their substance of choice once again. The truth is they are still a processed food addict (or alcoholic)—the disease of addiction still has to be treated on a daily basis.

Once a processed food addict, always a processed food addict.

A quick note on vegetarianism. If someone chooses to be vegetarian, that is their personal choice. A common pattern among potential processed food addicts starts with them announcing they are vegetarian. That is not a problem in quite a few cases. However, as treatment and recovery continue, some of these individuals go down the vegetarian path because they believe if they eat meat, they will put on too much weight. So vegetarianism is another method of control. Remember, a processed food addict will do almost anything rather than put on weight. However, as the disease progresses down the road, they will ingest heavy amounts of junk food under the guise of vegetarianism, which may inevitably lead to bingeing uncontrollably on processed foods, if they are a real processed food addict.

Once again, to thine own self be true. Anyone who is a vegetarian with core values of abstaining from meat products may use vegetarian protein in weighed amounts.

Ultimately, in recovery, the processed food addict moves beyond the processed food (how much or what they are eating), the body image, and the weight loss or gain, and is placed in a position of neutrality, with a new attitude toward processed food where they react sanely and normally. Now they are not fighting the processed food or avoiding temptation anymore, so long as their disease is treated on a daily basis.

The most important thing to note in treating processed food addiction is we eliminate processed foods. Below is a preliminary baseline plan for eliminating processed foods, where a potential processed food addict begins. Just that simple. At the end of the day, a recovered processed food addict will be food-obsession free.

Once again I would like to reiterate, this is a baseline prescription for eliminating processed foods. Recovery from the disease of processed food addiction over time is individualized with your qualified addiction specialist. The disease of processed food addiction may be the same, but it manifests differently in each person.

Preliminary Baseline for the Elimination of Processed Foods

The primary step in treating the disease of processed food addiction is to eliminate processed foods, while also weighing the quantities of non-processed foods ingested.

Men, please see the information at the end of this section.

BREAKFAST	LUNCH	DINNER	BGS (Blood Glucose Stabilizer)
Protein cooked 4 oz	**Protein cooked** 4 oz	**Protein cooked** 4 oz	**Dairy** 8 oz *or* **protein** 2 oz
Fruit 6 oz	**Raw salad** x 1 serving 8 oz	**Cooked vegetables** x 1 serving 10 oz	**Fruit** 6 oz
Carbohydrate 6 oz cooked whole grains *or* 8 oz cooked complex carbs	**Carbohydrate** 6 oz cooked whole grains *or* 8 oz cooked complex carbs	**Carbohydrate** 6 oz cooked whole grains *or* 8 oz cooked complex carbs	
Dairy 8 oz non-fat products (<.01% fat)		**Fats** 1 tbsp (15 ml) per day	

A Basic List of Non-Processed Food Products

This a basic list of non-processed food products to be used in the preliminary stages of eliminating processed foods.

Protein

1 serving (cooked) = 4 oz of beef, lamb, pork, veal, chicken, fish, shellfish, turkey; or 2 large eggs

Protein for vegetarians (before cooking): 1 serving = 8 oz tofu or 6 oz tempeh; or 8 oz beans and legumes

Fruit

1 serving = 6 oz of apple, all berries (strawberry, blueberry, raspberry, cranberry), apricot, cantaloupe, grapefruit, kiwifruit, lemon, lime, mandarin orange, nectarine, orange, passion fruit, peach, pear, pineapple, plum, rhubarb, tangerine, watermelon

Salad

1 serving = 8 oz

Cooked Vegetables

1 serving = 10 oz of artichokes, asparagus, beans, beets (beetroot), bok choy, broccoli, brussels sprouts, cabbage, carrots, cauliflower, celery, chicory, Chinese cabbage, cucumber, eggplant, endive, escarole, fennel, kale, lettuce (romaine, iceberg, Boston, butter), mushrooms, mung beans, okra, onions, parsley, peppers, pimentos, radishes, rutabaga, sauerkraut, snow peas, spinach, sprouts, tomatoes, turnips, water chestnuts, watercress, zucchini

Note: Salad serving and cooked vegetable serving may be interchanged (e.g., cooked vegetables at lunch and salad at dinner time).

Carbohydrates

Whole grains (cooked): 1 serving = 6 oz amaranth, barley, brown rice, brown basmati rice, buckwheat, grits, millet, oat bran, quinoa, rye, teff, steel-cut oats, or oats groats

Complex carbohydrates and starches (cooked): 1 serving = 8 oz beans (kidney, black, etc.) and legumes, winter squash (acorn, butternut, Hubbard, spaghetti or noodle squash, pumpkin), potato (yellow, red, white, sweet yams).

Dairy

1 serving = 8 oz non-fat (<.01% fat) product (skim milk, non-fat yogurt, non-fat soy milk)

Note: If you have an allergy to dairy, substitute 2 oz of protein.

Oils, Salad Dressings, and Accompaniments

1 serving (per day) = 1 tbsp (15 ml) of fats and oils (olive, canola, vegetable), Duke's mayonnaise (known as a clean brand of mayonnaise).

This one serving can be divided over breakfast, lunch, and dinner, throughout the day.

Sauces

1 serving (per day) = 1 tbsp (15 ml) of ketchup, salsa, mustard, horseradish, red wine vinegar, balsamic vinegar, dill pickles

Check that the ingredient list does not include processed, synthetic foods—artificial colorings or flavorings—or sweeteners.

Herbs, Seasonings, Spices

Herbs and Spices will be *your best friends* in recovery from processed food addiction, serving several purposes in cooking. They are used to enhance the natural flavors of food and to add a range of flavors from the natural sweetness of food to the kick of heat.

Bragg's Liquid Aminos, sea salt, pepper, mustard, cinnamon, salsa, red wine vinegar

Be wary of natural and artificial flavorings, and be sure that the herbs, seasonings, and spices are free of starch, hidden sugars, and so on. Consistently check ingredients, as products are inclined to change their ingredients.

Condiments

2 servings (per day) = 2 tbsp (30 ml) of either salsa or yogurt

Broth

1 serving (per day) = 8 oz (250 ml) Clean or homemade beef, chicken, or vegetable broth

Guidelines for Men

Please *increase* **protein** in **breakfast**, **lunch**, and **dinner** servings as follows:

Fish or poultry: add 2 oz (cooked)

Red meat: add 1 oz (cooked)

Eggs: increase to 3 large eggs

Tofu: increase to 12 oz (before cooking)

Please *increase* **lunch** servings as follows:

Add 1 **fruit** serving and 1 **carbohydrate** serving

Please *increase* **oils**, **salad dressings**, and **accompaniments** as follows:

Increase to 2 tbsp (30 ml) per day

Suggestion: divide among two or three meals throughout the day.

CHAPTER ELEVEN

Stories of Recovery

Processed food addiction as a branch of addiction is only just recently being discussed globally, as the manifestations of processed food addiction are many and varied. In classifying a person as a processed food addict, there is a huge amount of misunderstanding, ignorance, and bewilderment in this world that comes from people whose reactions are in contrast to that of a processed food addict. The paradigm of the phases of processed food addiction can help us here, as we can break it down a bit more.

Those in the early stages, up to the social and/or emotional eaters, are not bothered by how much they eat. They have a choice to either consume processed foods or not.

The next phases, up to crossing the line, are what I would class as *problem eaters* and *hard eaters*. Their physical and mental states may be impaired or deteriorating, causing them to die before their appointed time. But this person *can* stop or moderate their processed food consumption if they have adequate reason to do so. A new job offer, becoming pregnant, getting married, or a medical professional's help can become influential in stopping or moderating food usage, although it may be challenging, and they may need continued medical attention to carry it out. These are examples of what can influence a person using their logic to stop or moderate their processed food consumption.

The next stage is the most challenging when it comes to the diagnosis and classification of addiction. When I speak of processed food addiction, I am talking about the person who has tried every method conceivable to control, moderate, or stop their consumption of processed foods. Yes, this person is in the minority. In fact, this is what makes it so challenging to differentiate the *real* processed food addict (severe) from the processed food abuser.

In today's society, the psychiatric and psychological models have made a pathway to treating individuals whose experiences are somewhat different from those of real (severe) processed food addicts. Thus, when it comes to the real addict, these methods do not hold up over the ensuing months or years. Even more disheartening is that the real processed food addict is by far in the minority. They see others get well by methods they try to employ, but the effectiveness of these methods does not hold up over time—the real addicts are powerless to enact these same methods themselves. Or if they do, their lives are still quite miserable; they just eliminate the processed foods, changing nothing else, and finally they go back to the one source of ease and comfort they know only too well.

It is worth mentioning that even though a non-PFA may stop ingesting processed food for many months or even years, they are still similar to other people. However, in my professional and personal experience, I wholeheartedly affirm that when a real PFA ingests any processed food, their reaction is different from everybody else's. Something happens both physically and mentally that makes it almost impossible for them to stop. A colleague used the analogy of someone who is allergic to a wasp sting. One sting, even decades after the first allergic response to a wasp sting, causes a reaction that is worse than the first.

I have introduced these final case studies merely as illustrative of the truth that processed food addiction does not care about one's age, profession, or methods to control one's weight. The processed food addict is the master (though nearly always unconsciously) of their processed food status. While aiming to try to fix their condition, they are continually frustrating this achievement with thoughts and actions that cannot possibly harmonize with that end—a desire to ingest processed food just like others seem to do with ease. A processed food addict is suffering from a chronic disease that cannot be fixed. All these cases share one symptom in common: they cannot start ingesting processed food without the phenomenon of craving developing, which appears to be a huge contradiction to what they continually see all around them. The only known remedy I have to suggest, one which I support for severe processed food addicts, is complete abstinence.

Such cases could be multiplied and varied almost infinitely, but this is not necessary. You can, if you resolve to, take a look at your reflection in the mirror and introspectively look at the many attempts and failures in your own life of trying to control your consumption of processed food. Until this is done, external facts cannot serve as the ground for your reasoning. As those who trudge the road to a happy destiny say, recovery from addiction is an inside job, one day at a time.

Stories to Share

These patients have each willingly written their story and given their consent to be included in this book, believing their testimonies may give others hope that yes, you too can recover.

Can you identify with any of these stories? Look for the similarities, not the differences.

Julia's Expedition

Julia's story reiterates the potential processed food addict's powerlessness to beat the disease with the false belief that their weight is all that is wrong with them. Weight is the symptom of the primary cause. Julia used many methods of control, with the false belief that if she did this and did that, there would be an answer somewhere. If she could only fix her weight, then everything else would be great. More important to note is how her story demonstrates "once a processed food addict, always a processed food addict." Julia underwent weight-loss surgery and then unknowingly swapped the witch for the bitch: she replaced processed food with alcohol.

There are several types of weight-loss surgery; the majority of these aim to reduce the volume of the stomach so that the individual does not eat as much before feeling full. Julia could not ingest as much processed food as she used to without vomiting it back up. But once an addict, always an addict. The addict's brain still needs the "hit"—they chase the effect they get when they ingest, drink, or use. The effect is an experience of euphoria: all their troubles melt away, and their tension, anxiety, and loneliness subside.

As the disease of addiction progresses, the addict does not care what substance they use to get the hit. For Julia, alcohol did the trick, anesthetizing her brain for a time. However, the processed food addiction (her primary addiction) was still lurking subconsciously, just waiting for its chance to come back full throttle.

Julia says, "I could still ingest processed foods," albeit in much smaller amounts, which kept her processed food addiction alive. So she used the alcohol, but over time her ultimate craving for processed food was being ignited, until she did not have a choice. Then we see the patient showing up in clinic with not only a processed food addiction but a comorbidity of alcoholism (alcoholism and processed food addiction co-occurring). Interestingly enough, once I treated Julia's disease of processed food addiction, and she understood what the disease of addiction is about and how it manifested in her particular case, she could eliminate the substance and learn how to continually treat her disease of addiction on a daily basis.

> *My history with processed food goes back to my early childhood. Obsessing over and trying to control my weight, thinking that was the problem and strangely not connecting the weight to the processed food! It's only in later years, when I gained an understanding*

and knowledge about what was wrong with me, that I realized I have a disease (addiction). It has affected every aspect of my life—emotional, social, physical, and spiritual.

I ate because I had to. It was not a choice. I was out of control and driven to eat beyond physical comfort, crying as I stuffed the processed food in my mouth, unable to stop even when I wanted to. I was fighting an obsession and a compulsion beyond my ability to control.

I stole, lied, cheated, and manipulated to have processed foods. I isolated myself so I could eat and because I had little ability to interact with others in a healthy way. The damage to my personality was significant—with the ingestion of processed foods came a way of relating to others that was not healthy. I didn't mature and develop like my peers.

I was in 12 step programs for many years, starting at age twenty-nine. They dealt with food addiction and compulsive eating, and they all worked for a period of time, on and off. The trouble for me was they did not address the whole problem, just different aspects of the disease.

One fellowship might address the spiritual aspect, another might address the physical aspect, and another one the emotional aspect. But all aspects of the disease were not treated together.

I lost huge amounts of weight and thought that was the solution. I kept it off for many years, though I had slips along the way ... but still, the terrible fear of food and relapse always hung over my head.

An important point here is that Julia could not sustain permanent elimination of processed foods, let alone experience any relief from the physical and mental torture that comes with the addiction. This is another way the disease is still operative while being very subtle. Eventually a real processed food addict will ingest again and may end up in a mental institution or die. As you can read in the next part of Julia's history, the disease came back with a vengeance. The disease of addiction is progressive: it gets worse over time, never better.

> *I had a terrible plunge back into the disease full-time when I married late in life, and that led to a horrible six years of living in the insanity of the disease and its consequences.*
>
> *Terrible pain and crazy behaviors affected all I touched.*

Julia's life became quite unmanageable.

> *I made the decision at that time to have bariatric surgery (the sleeve), as I was gaining so much weight and nothing was working for me anymore. I had given up on recovery and trying to control the weight. I knew in my heart it was not the answer, but all I cared about at the time was how to stop the huge weight gains. I had gone from 149 lb. to 234 lb. (68 kg. to 106 kg.) in months and knew I would be 440 lb. (200 kg.) and not be able to work or function if I didn't do something drastic about my weight.*

We can see the hopelessness of the addict, who still believes "if only I could control this weight thing, then everything else will be fine."

> *I had a false sense of hope that this would be the answer, though deep in my heart I knew it wasn't.*
>
> *I didn't have much success because, of course, I could still ingest processed foods. I was in hospital for seven days, and after two days at home, I stole my stepson's chocolate out of his room and ate ice cream. The weight did not fall off me like it had done for others, as I still could not stop eating sugars and refined carbohydrates. Over the next two years, I probably dropped about 33 lb. (15 kg.) and kept it off by controlling my food intake with dieting and so on.*

My emotional and spiritual health were suffering, with crazy acting out, crying, distorted thinking, and blaming others for my problems and pain.

I also started to drink alcohol, and that started to become a problem [comorbidity was emerging]. I had added alcohol to processed food and I was terrified. I was obsessing on the way home from work about stopping to get a bottle of wine; I would have one glass and be drunk, then it was two glasses. My husband was very worried about this, but I kept minimizing the impact it was having. I had three small car accidents related to the drinking (backing into cars as I was driving out of my driveway). I always used to take a glass of wine down the park with my dogs, so I could drink alone. I was hiding what and where I was drinking, just as I did with the processed foods.

I really was at the end of myself and prayed for God to show me something new. I thought I had tried it all.

She had reached the stage of hopelessness.

Nothing I had done before worked anymore. God answered that prayer by sending my way a professional addictionologist and a fellowship that addressed the disease in all areas of my life by using the 12 steps to recover and stay recovered.

Not cured but recovered.

Julia understood through treatment what was going on; all these years she had not been bad, insane, a gluttonous pig, out of control, and so on. She suffered from the disease of addiction. No 12 step model can be sustained over time unless the addict understands they have a disease. It cannot be cured, but it can go into permanent remission if they follow their self-care plan, which includes the 12 step way of life for the majority of addicts.

I have worked hard in putting my recovery first, moved forward one day at a time, and am now a recovered processed food addict. Today, it's not about what food plan I'm on—I could not and cannot stick to any diet, any plan, with peace of mind long term. I was powerless. Today it's about recovery from a hopeless state of mind and body. Of course, I have a way of eating that is free of any processed food and I weigh my food so there is a clear boundary and I have enough fuel in my body to function within the 24 hours that present themselves. I am free today and no longer think or obsess about food, whether it be processed or not. I am free, and food is in its right place.

I treat my disease by attending meetings, doing my daily recovery practices, and staying close to God.

Today, I am a recovered processed food addict and I live a life of freedom where I am able to be of love and service to others.

Liz's Voyage

Food was always important to me. As a little kid, it soothed and comforted me. As I got older, food was not only a comfort but could numb me when I was feeling bad. It gave me something to do when I was bored, and it became an obsession that could distract me from just about everything else that was going on in my life.

Numb me, anesthetize me, hijack my brain: these actions all have the goal of chasing the effect. Here Liz learns early on that she must have the processed food to feel better.

The addict spends their life chasing this effect. That is the feeling and release they get when ingesting the substance. As time goes on, the processed food addict needs more and more of the substance to get the same effect they chased in earlier years. Tolerance increases, needing more and more of the substance (processed food) to achieve satiation or the desired effect—that is, to feel good, or preferably, not to feel at all. The withdrawal symptoms—depression, anxiety, stress, headaches, and so on—decrease once the processed food is ingested, even if only for a little while.

This is a good place to bring up different substances and their effects, specifically, processed food, which is the least understood. You see, when an alcoholic drinks alcohol, they can get drunk, pass out, or black out for several hours, overnight, or, in a minority of cases, days. It is similar with narcotics (depending on what narcotic is taken). When taking substances, the addict typically passes out rather than falls asleep naturally. When this happens, the brain is in a state that's analogous to being anesthetized, rather than actually asleep.

However, the processed food addict may ingest so much that they cannot physically get off the couch. They may doze off for a couple of hours, but unfortunately this substance (processed food) does not have effects as long-lasting as other substances. So, before long they are up again at the fridge, or in the cupboard, looking for their next hit. This is where the addict may start to look for something stronger, such as over-the-counter meds, or take up gambling, smoking, or drinking, or take on a relationship, with the added benefits of sex, to fill up the hole in the soul, so they feel wanted, needed, loved, and so on. Anything to make them feel better, or preferably, not feel or think at all.

As Liz's story goes on, we can see the progression of the disease of addiction. Of note is the relapse. Like any disease, if it is not treated on a daily basis, slips and relapses will always ensue. The denial creeps back in ever so subtly, and once again we think, "Well, perhaps I am not as bad as I thought I was." Blessedly, Liz's disease continues to stay in remission.

> *As a kid, I was a normal weight. I treated food as a substance to make me feel better but didn't have access to anything other than what Mom cooked and prepared for us. I was fairly active, playing outside a lot and playing a bit of sports at school. During my teens, I didn't pay much attention to my body; it did what it needed to do and got me where I wanted to go. I rode my bike to and from school and was quite slender.*

I left home at nineteen to go to university and I lived on my own for my first year. I was very lonely—it was the first time I'd ever been away from my family. I started eating more sugary, processed foods for comfort, but I still did a lot of exercise, walking a lot as I couldn't afford a car.

My four years at university were difficult. I had a lot of friends but felt very lonely, and the adult world confused and frightened me. Although I used processed food to comfort myself, it was early days in my disease and I wasn't exhibiting many outward symptoms such as excess weight. What I did feel was isolated and cut off from everyone else. My emotions would swing wildly from elation to terrible lows.

My weight began to increase when I started working full-time after university. I'd bought a car and was driving to and from work instead of walking and catching public transport. I went on my first diet when I was about twenty-four or twenty-five. It was the F-Plan—lots of fiber. I loved it, as I made lots of muesli with dried fruit! A year or two later, I tried a commercial diet where I bought their meals. I think I weighed about 165 lb. (75 kg.) at the beginning; they measured my wrist and told me I could weigh 136 lb. (62 kg.), which I thought sounded great. I'd weighed 143 lb. (65 kg.) when I finished high school and throughout my years at university.

By the time I was twenty-eight, my weight had increased again. I'd stopped weighing myself after I reached 172 lb. (78 kg.), as I just didn't want to know. By this stage, I'd realized that for me, it wasn't just about finding the right diet; I was using food differently from the people around me.

I joined my first 12 step program—Overeaters Anonymous (OA)— and in the first two years, I dropped down to 143 lb. (65 kg.) and stayed between 143 lb. and 148 lb. (65–67 kg.) for about eight years. Over this time, my career progressed, and I changed jobs a few times. I started recognizing patterns in my work behavior. I'd get a new job and work really hard, and deal with the stress by eating, and I'd put on weight. Then I'd get serious about my recovery work and start working with a new sponsor or going through the 12 steps again. And my weight would drop, and my stress levels would even out. But I'd get tired of that job and I'd start looking for the next step, the next promotion.

As my career progressed, my income naturally increased. I had problems managing money, often spending more than I could afford. The 12 step program had been very helpful in addressing my food issues, so I joined Debtors Anonymous to address my spending. It was very helpful, and the members were so supportive.

When I was thirty-seven, I met the man who would become my husband. We had a long-distance relationship for the first year, as we didn't live in the same country. After he moved to Australia, we sold the two-bedroom unit I'd lived in to be closer to my work and we bought a three-bedroom house.

I started to recognize how much I was using alcohol.

My job as usual was stressful, and I now had stepsons living in a different country. After one of our visits to New Zealand, I went home to Australia, knowing I needed to address the problems that alcohol and sugar were becoming for me. Although I was still attending OA and the 12 steps were really helpful, the food plan of eating moderately didn't seem to be helping me anymore.

Note the comorbidity—alcohol *and* processed food.

I found another 12 step program—Food Addicts Anonymous (FAA). They suggested a weighed and measured food plan and abstaining from all forms of sugar, flour, and wheat. While I thought at the time that was a little extreme, I also thought maybe something this extreme was what I needed.

> For three years, I followed the FAA food plan and continued to attend OA meetings, as there were no face-to-face FAA meetings in Australia at that time. My weight dropped to 137 lb. (62 kg.), the lowest I had ever weighed as an adult. I was delighted. But really, I was just controlling my weight using a food plan. Although I was a member of a 12 step fellowship, looking back now, I can see that I fitted my recovery into my life. I didn't fit my life into my recovery.
>
> It wasn't my highest priority—my career was.

Here, Liz is using her work to stay in denial about having an addiction. The addict seems to think, "If I can keep my job, then there can't be too much wrong with me. I may have a *little* weight and alcohol problem, but I'm nowhere as bad as those drunkards in the park, or my two work colleagues who are at least 50 lb. (22 kg.) overweight."

As addiction specialists are becoming more attuned to symptoms of the disease of addiction, the label *high-functioning addict*, or HFA, is being used. Typically this person is in denial about any substance abuse; they hide it under a smoke screen and cunningly turn the question back onto the person querying them: "I'm okay, what's wrong with you?" An addict will go to any lengths to not be questioned, challenged, or held accountable, unless it suits them, of course—once again, keeping them in denial. As you will continue to see in Liz's story, work and career came first, and as long as she could keep it going, who was going to judge her? Once again, if the person is a real processed food addict, there will come a time and a day where they will ingest again.

> I picked up processed food again in 2008. I kidded myself that it wasn't that bad. I didn't eat chocolate initially—I ate white chocolate and that didn't count (!!!). The level of justification and rationalization that I employed was significant. After abstaining from sugar, flour, and wheat for three years, my descent into active addiction was fast and horrible. I couldn't drive to work without stopping at least twice to buy and consume something before I

arrived at work. Often, I'd leave my workplace and drive to a local supermarket to stock up on things to get me through the day, the morning, or the afternoon. I spent huge amounts of money on binge foods.

The following year, I changed jobs again, to a more senior position at a different organization. My huge consumption of processed food continued. I was horribly ashamed of my weight gain—within a couple of months, I'd surpassed the heaviest I'd ever weighed. During this period, my weight topped out at 216 lb. (98 kg.).

I tried to return to FAA and follow their food plan, but I couldn't stick to it. I'd manage a week or so and then pick up again. I didn't realize at the time that I was propelled exclusively by self-will, and all the willpower and self-determination in the world couldn't stop me from putting chocolate in my mouth. However, I did get involved in the program again, and my sponsor told me that a person from the USA was coming to Australia and would be conducting a retreat in Brisbane in February 2013.

I was able to attend that retreat and it was the beginning of recovery for me, although it took another twelve months before I was able to abstain from processed foods. I found a fellowship of processed food addicts in Brisbane and was able to keep in touch with them. They encouraged me and demonstrated the miracle of living in recovery and following the 12 steps.

I returned to Brisbane the following year in February 2014 and asked someone to sponsor me. I spent a week in a rehabilitation setting for processed food addiction in Australia in March 2014, learning to live abstinently, and started to eliminate all forms of processed food. That's when I started to understand that my weight, my spending, and my workaholism were only symptoms of my disease, and that finding the right diet, food plan, or spending plan, or dealing with work-related stress, were not the answers for me. I learned how to start treating my disease.

> *Nine months later, in February 2015, I picked up processed food again, but thankfully it didn't develop into a full-blown binge. With a lot of rebelliousness, I got back on track and recognized I hadn't made my recovery my number-one priority—again!*

The addiction must be addressed in order for the processed food addict's disease to stay in remission.

> *I used to think I had problems with food, money, and work and I just needed to find the right 12 step fellowship with the right spending plan and food plan. Today, I recognize that my disease of processed food addiction does not distinguish between a professional and a non-professional, whether one earns the minimum wage or hundreds of thousands of dollars. For me as a processed food addict, ingesting any form of processed food brings me to my knees and I become self-absorbed and self-obsessed, filled with self-will. And so unhappy.*
>
> *Today, I have been eliminating processed foods (abstaining) for more than three years. I've moved countries and downsized my career and my life. I have a job I enjoy that doesn't have the high profile and big pressures I used to think I thrived on. My life today is small and manageable. My recovery is my highest priority. My family is my next priority. And my career comes third—sometimes further down the list. Most of the time today I am happy, joyous, and free, and so grateful that I have a solution to living, while my addiction to processed food stays in remission one day at a time.*

Lee's Odyssey

> *My first memory of bingeing was when I was eight. It was Christmas Day and I had eaten so much, I needed to vomit in the toilet. I don't remember too much more until I was eleven. I used to sneak into the kitchen in the dark, take the tin with chocolate cake down off the shelf and slice off slivers of cake, hoping people would*

not notice I had been there. I would wash it down with milk, hiding between the fridge and the wall so no one would see me. It was so hard to control how much cake I ate.

At the age of fourteen, I was at boarding school and my eating was out of control.

I would put my head in my locker, eating as many cookies as possible in the short time I had to do so, pretending I was looking for something. I lived to eat. My grandmother would visit me at school and all I could think about was what goodies she would bring me. I was by now putting on massive amounts of weight.

By age sixteen, I started my binge-starve cycle. I took diet tablets (speed) to control my bingeing, then I would come off them and binge. To control my weight, I went on crazy diets, joined Weight Watchers, bought Jenny Craig, tried hypnotism, purged, and exercised, just to name a few ways I tried to control my ingestion of processed food.

As time went on, I needed to eat larger amounts of processed food and I would eat for longer periods of time. I'd put muesli into a bowl, eat half of it, and then top it up again and again and again. In the end, having no idea how much muesli I'd eaten, I could tell myself I had only had one bowl. Consuming alcohol was a way I could get a quick hit (straight to the brain), so I began to drink excessively and binge at the same time. In my mind, this would control the weight.

Note, once again, the comorbidity. This is typical in the processed food addicts I treat, most of whom get "sober" or "clean" before they realize that their imbibing processed food is much more dangerous than just a "problem."

When this didn't work I would simply eliminate food groups (dieting again), but I would fool myself that I was being healthy. I became health obsessed, eating only organic food and so-called healthy food. I was still simply controlling my weight, which I managed to do for about seven years.

I was white-knuckling the whole time and getting sicker and sicker in my thinking. I would also undertake severe cleanses (e.g., drinking copious amounts of saltwater), so I would have diarrhea and not eat anything at the same time as part of my health regime, but, again, it was a way to control my weight. None of this worked for me, and by the age of fifty-eight, I was just getting sicker and sicker ... still thin, but very sick, and it was getting harder and harder to control my food.

We can note Lee's disease progressing here with her words "it was getting harder to control my food," and what comes next is that life becomes quite unmanageable.

My life was completely unmanageable. It was like living a double life, pretending everything was okay on the outside and that I had it all together. But all I could think about was food, what I could or couldn't eat, how I was going to stay thin, what I looked like, what people thought about me. I would buy a particular food (healthy, of course) and tell myself I would have it with coffee at home. No way was this going to happen, as I would have eaten it before I turned on the ignition. My mental health was deteriorating, and my thinking had become so distorted that it was becoming impossible to be in my skin.

More often than not, the processed food addict leads two lives. One they want the outside world to see, where they present as happy-go-lucky and everything is okay. They build upon this alter ego, seeming responsible, confident, and reputable at work. Their friendships and family life are presented as enviable to those they befriend over the years. This is the persona they want the world to see. However, their frequent travels are actually fictitious, and they lead a double life, hiding how much they ingest, where they ingest, when they ingest.

Having hundreds of excuses at the ready for why they have put on weight, why they can't attend a certain family function, why they have taken off more mental health days or sick days at work over the last twelve months.

Then in come the professionals, who question why this person acts this way, doing all they can to help them, only to find the processed food addict rationalizing again why they did such-and-such. Very rarely will a processed food addict tell *anyone* the whole truth, let alone follow their advice. Not surprising that medical and health specialists are disconcerted when the patient, time after time, comes in with yet another rationalization or self-justification as to why they did not stick to that diet or why they did not follow their advice.

> *This was my disease progressing.*
>
> *Over the years, I was diagnosed with depression and put on antidepressants. I was diagnosed with obsessive-compulsive disorder and I had general anxiety. I was medically diagnosed with these disorders, but I also did a lot of self-diagnosing, trying to work out what was wrong with me and searching for the answers.*
>
> *In my early twenties, I went to Overeaters Anonymous (OA) because deep down I knew something was wrong. I was in and out of OA for many years, also trying other 12 step fellowships for food addiction (e.g., RFA [Recovery from Food Addiction Anonymous] and CEA-HOW [Compulsive Eaters Anonymous–Honest, Open-Minded, Willing]).*
>
> *I went to AA nearly fourteen years ago to address my alcohol addiction, but I kept using processed food. I was not getting well, as I said before; I was getting sicker and sicker and pretending in AA that I was living a spiritual way of life and all was good with me.*
>
> *At the age of fifty-eight, on October 9, 2015, I started to learn about the disease of processed food addiction and how it had manifested*

in my life. I learned that if I ingest processed food—even one crumb—I will trigger the phenomenon of craving and I will need more and more processed food.

It is also a biochemical disease, meaning that if I ingest processed foods, it makes my brain very sick and my thinking becomes distorted.

From that day forward, I started to treat my disease of processed food addiction, and it has been in remission ever since. It is not a psychological disease. I cannot blame my family or events in my life for my addiction. I ingest processed food because I have the disease of processed food addiction.

Now, in recovery, I do not crave processed foods—I simply eat to fuel my body, so I can get on with what I need to do in a day. I do not need to control my weight. I am not as obsessed with how I look and worried about what people think of me. My mental health has improved remarkably, and the distorted thinking that used to torture me is not a problem for me today. I feel spiritually well and practice living spiritual principles in my life. Twisted relationships are being untwisted and I quite like myself today. I have family in my life that love me, and I love them.

My work life does nothing but surprise me—never in a million years would I have thought I would be doing what I am doing. It is amazing work and I get to be of service to many people. I can be there for others today, because it is not always about me. I am learning I am human, it is normal to make mistakes, and I will never be perfect (this was a big one for me, but it is starting to sink in). I don't get angry like I used to, and if I do, it shifts very quickly. I feel joy and peace today, and I feel so grateful because I know what's wrong with me, as I live in the solution. I don't have to fix myself anymore because there is nothing wrong with me. I simply have a disease.

It has not been easy, as I have spent many years being sick in the disease of processed food addiction. I needed to be treated by an addictionologist, who, after treating me, helped me to find a 12 step program (Processed Food Anonymous) to continue my recovery from this disease. I have recovered, and life is vastly different. Treating this disease daily has become the norm for me and I am so grateful because my life is immensely different. I will be treating this disease one day at a time for the rest of my life, as I will never be cured, but I wouldn't have it any other way. Living life without a substance is the best and it can only get better.

Throughout all the years I list below, I was continually seeking all types of counselors, therapists, and medical professionals to fix me. No one was at fault; they just did not know I was suffering from a disease of processed food addition. They just thought I was a food abuser and that behavior methods among other control measures would fix me. I know today, you cannot fix an addict. Just like an endocrinologist cannot fix someone who has diabetes. But my disease can and has been treated.

1964—First memory of a binge—all through primary school I felt fat and different

1972—High school as a boarder and starting to put on lots of weight

1974—Began a starving and bingeing cycle

1982—Tried OA

1990—Tried AA

1993—Tried Al-Anon

Another try of OA somewhere in between here

2003—AA

2009—CEA-HOW

2009—OA again

2010–2015—controlling my weight—such hard work

> *2015—tried RFA*
>
> *2015—started working with an addictionologist*
>
> *2016—got into PFA, where I heard the solution to my disease of processed food addiction*
>
> *2018—Still abstinent with peace of mind, going into my fourth year of recovery. My disease of processed food addiction is staying in remission. This is the norm for me today.*

Jacinta's Journey

> *When I reflect back on my earliest memory of having an eating problem, it is when I was in grade 6 and my cousin was in grade 7. Our classrooms were separated by a playground. I can clearly see her walking across the playground with a fruit roll-up to give to me at break time. In detail, I remember it being pink and purple, and was an apple and blackcurrant flavor. Thinking about ingesting the fruit roll-up when I was a young girl, I remember that sense of Ahh, a letting go, a feeling that "everything is going to be okay."*

This is the effect, or hit, that every addict knows only too well; this is what the processed food addict chases over and over again. Something, anything, to hijack the brain and save it from facing reality.

> *How quickly that changed for me; soon, I no longer got that relief when I ingested processed foods, as my disease quickly progressed.*
>
> *For me, I have been obese as long as I can remember, right from when I was in primary school. The shame I carried around with the weight was huge. Right from primary school, I would avoid interacting socially in daily life tasks that made me uncomfortable, and this only progressed into high school and early adulthood. For example, I would have excuses for why I couldn't engage in physical activity class, accompanied by notes I had forged pretending to be my parents, as I was too uncomfortable to have fat wiggling if I*

ran. I would not go out with friends. I did not want them to see me eat, as I told myself they would judge my eating and my weight, and I thought this meant they were judging me.

Note the devilish addict personality (*dap* is Jacinta's name for her disease) coming in here, so very, very subtly. "Everyone *will* judge me in regards to what I eat and how fat I am." This is the beginning stages of a potential processed food addict, as the voice stays hidden and quite deceptive, blaming Jacinta for having a weight problem. Yes, the majority of people may have a weight or food problem. However, there is a minority who, like Jacinta, no matter what they do, will never be able to ingest processed foods normally. As soon as they ingest the processed food, it sparks off the phenomenon of craving to ingest more.

Next, Jacinta's disease progresses quite rapidly.

But, for me, when my disease really accelerated was when I hit year 10, aged fifteen. One of my teachers identified me as being depressed and forced me to see the school counselor. The disease loved this! Not only did people pay me special attention, I could get out of classes I didn't like and, most importantly, felt that was the answer, explaining why I felt different from my peers.

Jacinta is now becoming a pro when it comes to hiding her disease. I know, and every processed food addict I work with knows, deep, deep down inside, there is something different about us. We can't in the early stages put our finger on it, but we intuitively know. I wonder whether that is why we spend a lifetime (until we get well) trying to prove we are just like other people. Food for thought (pun intended).

From age fifteen, the negative mind really caned me into believing I was only worth anything if my grades were, at the minimum, distinction standard. I strived to be the top of my class—this included not helping my friends and lying that I didn't know the answer

> *so that I could get the leg up. The fear and anxiety I had around achieving these marks had me studying all night and waking up at the crack of dawn to study. Friends dropped off, as studying and ingesting (to ensure I had fuel to study, as my mind told me) was all I could fit into a day.*

Ah, Jacinta. The disease is now using study to hide the reality and to give her believable excuses to tell those around her. Who could judge Jacinta for being obese if her grades were at this standard? Once again, another form of escape: "You can't judge me. Look at what I am doing at university!"

> *I had daily thoughts and ideas of wanting to end my life, as I thought I would always fail and not reach the standards I set myself. At times, I couldn't see the point to even try.*
>
> *At the end of my year 12 exams, I broke down. I would wake up crying in panic and being unable to function. The ingesting went from bingeing to starving like a yo-yo and the guilt associated with this was HUGE, as I no longer had the excuse in my mind that I had to ingest to ensure I had the brain power to study.*
>
> *This was when I found myself being taken by my parents to a local GP to fix me.*

Nothing is broken in the processed food addict. The person is just suffering a disease of addiction that *can* be treated.

> *I started on antidepressants and marked the commencement of my career with one-on-one psychologist appointments. Neither of these treatments worked, despite eight years doing both alongside medical recommendations. Rather, I believe they enabled me to get to the age of twenty-five before completely reaching rock bottom rather than earlier on.*
>
> *So, at the age seventeen, the disease was familiar with using processed foods, study, and antidepressants and depending on my family and psychologists.*

Jacinta now had a familiar pattern of denial, which was only going to continue to be stuffed down further, as she did not want to ever know the truth or to admit it to herself.

Who wants to be a processed food addict? Come on, let's get honest. Yeah, maybe an emotional eater, a problem eater, a food addict, a compulsive overeater, a chocoholic, a sugarholic, and so on. But not a processed food addict, *ugh!*

I have heard processed food addicts say, "K-L, I call this my dirty little secret that no one will *ever* know about."

I find this very sad, as I know only too well the magnitude of this disease and its power to keep a potential addict in denial. Using study and antidepressants, having family and health professionals and later on relationships or even pets, anything for me to try to appear normal when it comes to ingesting processed food.

> *It then stepped up a gear and brought in distorted sexual relationships with anyone who gave me a second of attention, as the self-esteem I had at this point was tiny. These attentions boosted my self-esteem temporarily and then led me back to ingesting, as I felt remorseful for my actions.*

> *My alcohol intake also accelerated to the point where I would enjoy a Baileys and full-cream milk in the mornings and port every evening. I also had the perception that I suffered from constant headaches and pain, which led me to most days needing medications with codeine, which also had muscle relaxants in them. I would take two over-the-counter pain relievers with nil effect by this point, along with other medications.*

> *The disease continued to pull in a bachelor's degree, two online courses, getting married, a master's degree, buying a house, and owning two dogs as ways to deny myself the realization that I had a chronic and fatal disease of processed food addiction, and attempted to give me the illusion I was doing well and everything was okay.*

Once again, the disease is progressing—here is the disease now pulling, using anything and everything to keep Jacinta in denial and believing that now that she has qualifications, a house, and a pet, she appears normal to the rest of the world. In other words, Jacinta is externally displaying "Don't judge me for my weight or my food choices, as I am normal. I have and do just what everyone else does."

Now, this would be fine—and is fine for the majority of people—if Jacinta did not have the physiological craving, the allergy that compels her to ingest processed foods once she starts.

Non-PFAs do not experience withdrawal symptoms that increase in severity as they continue to ingest. They never experience the need to ingest, and for them it is absolute torture to continue ingesting processed foods past the point of fullness. When they have had enough, they stop.

But for Jacinta, not ingesting the processed foods is far more agonizing, as her brain has adapted to only functioning normally with processed foods.

> *I was in so much emotional pain inside, though. I hated myself and I was resentful and angry with everyone that walked near me, though I manipulated situations to portray "poor me" and how I was a saint trying to help others. What lies and manipulation. I now understand I was in a state of denial, though the disease at this point had me fooled too.*
>
> *I found my way into Processed Food Anonymous (PFA) at the age of twenty-five. It had been five months since I graduated university with my last degree, and I found I could no longer cope. I had put on 22 lb. (10 kg.) in one month as my bingeing increased to every day and my thought process was a) suicide or b) hypnotism.*

Here Jacinta is saying she had ingested enough and her way was not working anymore. Time had passed, there was no more study to distract or make excuses for her, and her life was becoming more and more unmanageable. I sometimes think this is how the universe works.

When we have had enough and are willing to have an open mind, people, places, and things are put into our lives in a positive way.

Here Jacinta's family member knew a little about food and addiction and suggested Jacinta try the 12 step approach. As the saying goes, when the student is ready the teacher appears. Coincidence? God working anonymously? Perhaps. But, gee, there are a lot of coincidences among the people I treat.

> *Luckily for me, I reached out to a family member who suggested a 12 step program. I had never considered that addiction could be my problem. I was so desperate that I went to a food 12 step fellowship that next week and kept going, as I knew there was no hope of me doing it by myself anymore. This food fellowship could not get me abstinent, as food was still largely a topic discussed and this would play in my mind all the time. Thankfully, within six months of being in a food fellowship, I went to a workshop where I heard a specialist (an addictionologist who treated processed food addiction) share about the disease of processed food addiction.*
>
> *For the first time in my life, I started to identify my problem.*

Jacinta is identifying here that she is neither alone nor different. Processed food addicts, like all persons with addiction, speak a language I have come to know as the Language of the Heart. They have their own special language. People with addictions can empathize with each other, love each other, and laugh with each other and at the many adventures their addiction has taken them on. They are what I call *insiders*.

Outsiders are what I call *earthlings* to my patients. They have not experienced the disease of processed food addiction, which makes it challenging for them to understand. Heaven knows, it was hard enough for us to come to terms with our disease, let alone someone who has never experienced it. Over time, though, the line slowly disappears and there is an understanding, a compassion, and more to the point, relief, as their loved one is finally getting help. The suffering they have watched and partaken in over many sleepless nights is now waning. Their loved ones, friends, colleagues, and so on are now smiling and seem to have come to an understanding underpinned by unconditional love. Analogous to those around someone with a disease, those who know an addict learn to love them unconditionally and to do what they can to help them to stay well and keep their disease of addiction in remission.

> She answered so many questions, but I still had a thousand more to ask. So, I commenced to work with her and started to treat my disease of PFA: eliminating processed food, becoming abstinent, starting working the steps, and looking at how the disease manifested in my life—that unmanageability.
>
> Now, I am eighteen months abstinent and sober, no longer taking antidepressants or the countless prescribed over-the-counter medications, or attending forever ongoing psychologist appointments. I am able to show up at a full-time job and be of service to others. With the help of God, the character defects that had me previously living in selfishness, fear, resentment, and dishonesty are being removed, and I am working toward a relationship with my family and partner that is on a loving basis and not manipulative, dysfunctional, and prideful.
>
> I am also finding the real Jacinta—who I am. I am learning that there is, and will continue to be, a lot of change in my life, a life that was hidden under the mask of processed food addiction.

Rob Remembers

> My first diet was when I was about eight. I ate three lettuce leaves with salt; I think I had seen this diet in a magazine. I also ran up and down a hallway twenty to a hundred times.
>
> The next diet I remember, I was about age sixteen. A boyfriend had told me I was fat, and I went on a calorie-counting diet. I had 800

calories a day and my friend in class drew a picture of me riding my bike with a calorie counting book under my arm. That was the theme of my life. I had a pink box with rewards inside it for when I achieved my end result after four weeks. I had creams and powders.

But the truth is, what really happened was I binged on bakery goods, vanilla slice being my top pick. I was fairly out of control with processed food at about this time, fifteen, sixteen, and seventeen, making creamed butter and sugar after school.

Comorbidity kicks in again here.

But around sixteen, I also discovered alcohol, and then at eighteen, I discovered drugs. I loved how these helped me to feel thin—I could use them to control my appetite. I didn't need to eat, and if I did, it would take away the high. Eating was for the weak. When I did eat, I was free to eat processed food because I didn't eat often, and I stayed slim. Not for long.

In my mid-twenties I was bigger, and by my late twenties I was quite big. I joined AA to arrest my binge drinking. I also went to OA and then to FA. I lost weight and felt very superior. I loved being slim again and I connected to a higher power. I loved AA. I began to get well. After almost two years in FA, however, I was angry and very controlling. I binged and began to purge with vomiting. I ate cheap food that was off and spoiled. I ate a large family-size chocolate bar followed by a pack of mint slices ... I could eat so much. When I tried to sleep, it was fitful, and my body was hot from all the food in me. I ate until my stomach hurt and then felt so very sad that I could not eat again until the food had gone through my system and I was hungry again. I longed to be hungry again so I could eat once more.

I went to a meditation course and was asked to put down (not eat) any addictive substances. I put down sugar for the ten-day retreat. After meditation, I did not pick sugar or wheat back up. For ten years, I ate healthy food AND binged on it too. I lived my life and all seemed well, pursuing my goals and dreams. But every day I looked to the food. Was it roast vegetables with hummus? Was it yogurt and dried fruit? Whatever food it was that day, I had to know that it was endless. I held off until 11 a.m. before I started to ingest, because I knew I could not stop after that. I would slowly graze and binge all day.

I became vegetarian and vegan for years, yet I eventually became thicker around the middle—this terrified me. I joined FAA, I lost weight, and became successful in the program.

But after almost two years, when people told me I was doing well, I felt a seething resentment swelling around inside of me, like a poisonous gas that seeped out the sides. I knew something was very wrong. I had been eating (non-processed) foods in an addictive way. I was controlling the little bit of food I was allowed with all of my might. I was tied up in knots about it. When I got on the scales I became so excited to see the number. If it was lower, I had a brilliant day. But something was still wrong. I just knew it. I was feeling bitter—black bitter inside. I didn't know why, and I didn't know that I didn't have to live like that. I had given up.

It is quite common for a set of scales to predict the day ahead for a processed food addict. The number can take on a life-or-death meaning. "If the number on the scales drops, even by half a pound, then that means I will have a good day. But! If the scale reads an ounce higher, then my day is shot—I'm doomed."

A lot of people (more often women than men) give power to the number on the scales. However, it does not interfere in their life the way it does for a processed food addict. Jumping on and off the scales 24-7, or whenever they feel like it, might be the dubious luxury of most people, but for a processed food addict, it can be deadly. Why? Once again, it gives the illusion that the processed food addict is responsible for their weight loss or gain. Loss means they can finally control it;

gain means they now have to lose it. Once again, the processed food addict is unable to control their weight via what they ingest, because sooner or later, they will ingest processed food, which leads inevitably to gaining weight. If we don't ingest processed food, we don't get fat; if we don't drink alcohol, we don't get drunk.

> *I knew I needed some processed or even non-processed food to use every day to cope with life. If I ate a lot of non-processed food (I mean a lot), I still felt like my brain was getting a kick. Whether it was a big pile of mustard or cinnamon. Whether it was vitamin C tablets with orange flavor. Whether it was green energy powder drinks. I swapped and changed ways to get my fix when the previous way made me sick.*

For the disease of processed food addiction to be ignited, the individual does not necessarily have to ingest processed foods. This is an important note to make, as it can be what keeps a lot of processed food addicts in denial far longer than they should have been. This is why in the preliminary stages of recovery, we commence with a plan of eliminating processed foods. As the recovery progresses, the processed food addict understands they cannot ingest processed foods or that action will lead once again down the black hole.

They may start to get bored or think they can do it now, thinking it is okay to ingest extra non-processed food. They might start off with having extra protein, extra fruit, extra rice, or oil or whatever. But always lurking in the back of the mind is the disease of processed food addiction. Once the addict begins in this nonchalant way, they start to think, "Well, I got away with that. Perhaps I am better now, and it will be different this time; therefore, I can control the rest of my food."

So they ingest low-fat yogurt, perhaps some rye bread or crackers. Then that may be okay for a couple of days or even weeks, and then before they know it, the mental twist kicks in and they start ingesting cookies, chocolate, and the like. The addict is once again in denial, believing falsely that "One day, somehow, I will be able to control and enjoy my ingestion of food," by which they always subliminally mean processed food control. Thinking they can now control and enjoy as much non-processed food as they want tells them they will one day be able to control and enjoy processed food forever. Well, for a severe processed food addict, this day will not arrive. Complete abstinence is the only way I know for a processed food addict to be free in body, mind, and spirit.

> *In this dark private state, I found an addictionologist. I hated everything she said, because I felt so challenged, but I wanted to be well. So, I tried what she said; I had nothing to lose. I immediately started to feel better; each day I got a little bit more trust.*
>
> *The worst thing for me was that this processed food addiction is not a recognized disease. And I felt like a liar and a weakling. But I watched the process of how it had worked in my life and I saw the disease standing alone.*
>
> *Today, after treatment, I operate free of my disease.*

Sheri's Crusade

> *My first memory involving food was when I was about five years old. I would hate getting my hair cut and would throw a fit every time. The only way they could get me to calm down was to give me the entire candy jar, which they sat on my lap, and I happily indulged in the candy as they cut my hair.*
>
> *My childhood memories involving food and weight consist of seeing Dr. Wolf every year for my annual checkup, and him telling me I had to lose weight. My parents were also overweight, so I watched their countless attempts at weight loss—Weight Watchers, the cabbage soup diet, liquid diets, more Weight Watchers ... I was always the fat kid in school and in my social groups. I loved to eat, especially junk food and particularly sweets. I always thought I just had a sweet tooth.*

Fast forward to my adolescent years, and in came the attempts at weight loss—Slim Fast or whatever the fad diet was at that time. In my teenage years, I was successful for the first time. I ate healthier and exercised, and it worked to an extent. However, I could never reach that ultimate goal weight I had in my mind—the weight where I imagined I would be pretty and popular and comfortable.

When I got to college, I was elated that I did not gain the "freshman 15." Instead, I waited until after my freshman year, then gained much more than fifteen pounds.

The "freshman 15" is the typical amount of weight (15 lb., or 7 kg.) a student gains in their first year of college.

College is also when I got drunk for the first time. I was never into alcohol that much, but I was curious what it felt like to be inebriated, so I set out on a mission one day and achieved it. I drank Jack Daniels Downhome Punch and was pleased with the effects. Unlike some other alcoholics, I was not off to the races with alcohol. Instead, I enjoyed the occasional drunk or buzz, but what I really sought was the effects of processed food.

Dare I say it, comorbidity is here again. This is a common underlying symptom of processed food addiction. Although, I was working with an alcoholic last week and as we were sharing about comorbidity, he said, "K-L, I'm a purebred," meaning he did not do drugs, processed food, gambling, or any other addiction—only alcohol.

I graduated from college (I was always a good student) and a couple years later met Steve online. I moved in with him within a few months. This was my first time on my own out of my parents' house and also my first relationship. This man was so much fun, carefree, attractive and most importantly, he was into me. But not into me enough that he was willing to commit to a monogamous

> *relationship. I wasn't happy with that, but I settled for it because I loved that an attractive man was giving me attention.*
>
> *What I didn't know when I met this man was that he was in his development of a pill addiction with some huffing on the side.*

Huffing is a type of substance abuse that involves inhaling fumes from toxic chemicals (for example, paint), which provide an intense high that *can* be easily obtained.

> *This is when I was introduced to opiates and a class of benzodiazepines (pain pills). Prior to that, I remember being prescribed Vicodin for some dental work, but I didn't take to them at that time. However, when Steve gave me a pill one night, I was in heaven. I melted into the mattress and slept like I had never slept before. All I felt was bliss, and the committee that had been in my head for so long—especially when I was trying to go to sleep at night—was pushed out by one little pill.*

The "committee" Sheri is referring to is the voice in her head, her odap, that says, "You are weak and pathetic. You'll never amount to anything. Surely everyone can control how much they eat and be thin. What's wrong with you? That's right, you're fat and lazy. You might as well go on and keep eating."

This committee is also known as the "itty-bitty shitty committee."

> *The progression of my pill addiction (predominantly benzodiazepines) started very slowly. Half a pill would do the trick and only on weekends ... maybe an evening here and there. At some point, half a pill wasn't cutting it any longer, so I upped it to one pill and the progression continued. Fast forward to the late stages of that process, and I was ordering a compound drug online that was far more potent than anything I could get from a local doctor or off the streets (with the exception of heroin). My life was in a shambles; planning, getting, and taking those pills consumed my world.*

> *Anything not to feel anxious or depressed, or face a panic attack. Those pills were like magic.*

> *At age twenty-eight, I found myself in a twenty-eight-day inpatient rehab. I couldn't believe that was me, that I was a drug addict. I ate my way through those twenty-eight days. Breakfast, lunch, dinner, and lots of snacks in between. Multiple portions at each meal, and my favorite was when they brought the candy out to sell. We weren't allowed to bring any food up to our rooms, but everyone did it.*

> *One day, I had bought some candy and tucked it in the back waistband of my pants to sneak it up to my room. As I was walking down the hallway, I felt the candy slip out and into the seat of my pants. I knew one of the counselors was standing in the room I had come from and I could feel her eyes on the back of me. I turned around to see her down the hallway, shaking her head as she said, "That dope fiend mentality…"*

Dope fiend is slang for "drug addict."

> *I was so embarrassed and humiliated. I had no idea just how far down my disease of processed food addiction would take me.*

> *Upon discharge from that rehab, I was given a prognosis of "guarded."*

Guarded refers to a probable outcome when a patient's recovery from her illness is in doubt.

> *They recommended I do an outpatient program, but I didn't think I needed that. I would be fine going to 12 step meetings and following the suggestions of getting a sponsor and working the steps. I was told to "grow where you're planted," so I tried both AA and NA and felt at home in AA, even though drugs were my thing.*

During this time, my eating continued to escalate more and more out of control. I would try a diet and couldn't stay on it for more than a day or two. My weight was rapidly increasing, and I was complaining about it to everyone I knew. One day, a coworker brought in an ad from a health magazine about food addiction classes and my ears perked up. I had heard of Overeaters Anonymous, but I was too embarrassed to go. I signed up for these classes and it turned out the woman who was teaching them was in another 12 step fellowship for food addiction. I quickly started that food plan and attending those meetings in addition to my AA meetings.

Things were progressing nicely (with the exception of my drug-addicted boyfriend).

Sheri is now free of all her addictive substances, including narcotics, alcohol, sugar, flour, and wheat. But she is still with a person who is addicted to drugs. In the recovery field we say, "If you are in the barber's shop long enough, you will get a haircut."

For the first time in my life I felt a freedom from the food and from these cravings that drove me to eat. I thought I had found the solution, and so I had for a period of time. I stayed abstinent for about a year as I continued to attend AA and RFA. I painfully ditched the boyfriend. I eventually got back on the food plan, but soon, a few years into sobriety, I noticed my anxiety was getting worse and my OCD-like symptoms were back. I just knew that I was one of those people who had a chemical imbalance in my brain and needed meds.

I told my AA sponsor my epiphany and she cautioned me about taking antianxiety or antidepressant medications. She suggested I seek therapy first to see if that helped. I reluctantly obliged and sought out a therapist who specialized in eating disorders. She was great! I totally believed in cognitive behavioral therapy: change the thought to change the feeling. It made sense!

> *I saw this therapist for a little while and felt better, so I stopped going to her.*
>
> *Not long after that I busted, with the processed food.*

Busted means she relapsed by slipping and picking up processed food again.

> *No matter what I tried, I could not get abstinent again.*
>
> *I went back to the therapist, thinking she could fix me, but it did not work this time. I was now convinced that I needed medication for my anxiety, so I went to a psychiatrist and told him I had heard about Effexor and would like to try that. He diagnosed me with OCD and gave me a script. The meds helped, my OCD diminished, and I eventually got my abstinence back.*

Here in Sheri's case we can see the multi-comorbid addiction diagnosis of alcoholism, drug addiction, and processed food addiction, plus the diagnosis of obsessive-compulsive disorder (OCD).

> *I stayed abstinent for about five years after that. I was the poster child for abstinence and food recovery. I learned I was a food addict—I had a label. I mostly attended RFA with some OA on the side.*
>
> *By this time, I had stopped attending AA because processed food was my primary addiction and I felt I needed to focus on those meetings. I also did not date or have any relationships during this period of abstinence. But toward the end of my five-year reign, I reconnected with the drug-addicted boyfriend Steve, who claimed he was sober now.*
>
> *Around the same time, I discovered coconut water, which I justified was clean because it was just water from a coconut.*

Here is the subtleness of the disease of processed food addiction. After five years of abstinence, Sheri justified it would be okay to have coconut water *because* it came from a coconut. The disease is cunning, baffling, and powerful. Look what happens next—the phenomenon of craving develops and Sheri passes through the well-known phases of bingeing. Coming out the other side, she feels guilty, hopeless, and full of regret, but promises to not ingest again, as she adds coconut water to the list of *can't haves*.

> *My eating grew out of control again, but I white-knuckled it and was determined to get and stay abstinent again. Steve and I had grown apart and I started a new relationship with another man who lived in my neighborhood, John.*
>
> *I was elated, and my food was under control. I would hang out with my neighbors, including John, while they drank, smoked, and ate merrily. But I stayed sober and abstinent. John would not commit to me, but like with Steve, I settled, even though deep down I was not okay with that.*
>
> *As this relationship and time went on, I gradually started messing around with food until I was full-blown bingeing on candy and fast food—anything I could get my hands on. I was completely defeated, so I went down south and stayed in a food addiction counselor's home to help me get back on track. When I got home, I lasted less than a month and busted again. Now I did not know where to turn, but I had seen my best friend get well from working with an addictionologist who specialized in processed food addiction. I had met this addictionologist several times but wanted nothing to do with her. I contacted her and so began my recovery.*
>
> *First of all, she helped me to understand how imperative it is to understand the disease of addiction in general and specifically my disease of processed food addiction. It was a relief to find out that I wasn't bad, just very sick, and that is what I had been suffering from all these years.*
>
> *As I commenced to grasp what the disease of processed food addiction is all about, she then helped me to see how it had manifested in my life. I stayed in the relationship with John even though I was*

> told it was not conducive to my recovery. I was also still friends with Steve. When things continued to go downhill with John, I brought in another man on the side to fulfill that sexual instinct that was so out of whack it wasn't funny.

Typically, a processed food addict will have had several relationships, be in a dysfunctional relationship, or be looking for another relationship to try to fill that hole in the soul that is left once processed food and other substances are eliminated. This side of the disease is addressed once the processed food addict is clean from all their substances. Only then can they comprehend how other people, places, and things have been masking the underlying addiction.

> By this time, I had also stepped down from my position at work into another role I had done previously; I was not able to perform the position from which I stepped down and I was barely able to perform the one I was trying to do.
>
> I finally hit a bottom where I realized I needed intensive inpatient treatment. My addictionologist encouraged me, so I agreed, and I stayed at a recovery house for a couple of months until I flew to Australia for an inpatient stay. Before the journey to Oz, my disease was still trying its best to be active, so I started to get treatment on a daily basis with the addictionologist.
>
> Life was not easy when I was a practicing addict, but it was even harder when the substances and other things were taken away. I had so many layers to my disease that I had to address them one at a time. I had eliminated the antidepressants and the antianxiety meds and the benzodiazepines. Then I eliminated the processed food, and lastly, I eliminated the men in my life, the sexual relationships, all with the specialist's help.
>
> I felt empty, scared, confused, emotional, depressed, anxious, and panicky at times. I would wake up every morning and my first thought was "shit" or "f**." I did not want to live, but for some

reason, I didn't go any further with suicide other than thinking about it and planning how I could do it. For the first time in my life, I knew there was hope for me.

I recall a period of about a week when the symptoms described above were so severe it felt like I was having a constant panic attack. I soon learned that these symptoms were a combination of consequences of the addiction—when I ingested—as well as withdrawal symptoms.

I continued to hold on to the older, sober, abstinent members at the 12 step fellowships telling me that they were once where I was and that it gets better. I didn't believe them, but again, I was too chicken to kill myself. So I trudged on, continuing to treat my disease, learning all I could about it and going through the 12 steps as they are outlined in the book Alcoholics Anonymous.

For the first time in my recovery, I started implementing those 12 steps and getting down to causes and conditions instead of just treating the symptoms of my disease (weight, processed food intake, anxiety, and so on). I was so used to using a person, place, or thing to deal with life, I had no idea how to live without using them.

I continued to work with this professional, who was able to help me look at myself and how my disease manifested in me, as I now understand it manifests differently in each addict. Very slowly, my life began to improve. One day, I noticed I wasn't waking up every morning with a feeling of dread and panic. I was able to function a little better at my job. I was experiencing that psychic change that is necessary for an addict to recover from this fatal malady.

More than eighteen months later, my life is unrecognizable from what it was before. At my job, I was able to go back to the position from which I had stepped down and I have begun to pursue a gift that God has given me with American Sign Language interpreting.

It is absolutely miraculous how God picked me up from the depths of despair, set my feet upon a rock, and rocketed me into the fourth dimension of existence.

This "fourth dimension of living" is a phrase that generally means the individual is now living in the spiritual world. Sheri knows she has a purpose in life, and daily she experiences peace of mind—the panacea of life. It cannot be taught or bought; it is only given and received by Grace.

It is not an easy journey; there have been many hurdles along the way, but I continue to treat my disease and die a little more to my self-centeredness each day. I do my best to implement all 12 steps in my life on a daily basis. I fall short many times, but because I am recovered and my disease is in remission, I have choices today, and I have the chance to keep practicing life without using a substance, person, place, or thing.

Today, it has gone from my head to my heart that I have a chronic illness—processed food addiction—which is similar to my alcohol and drug addiction, only the processed food addiction was very well hidden and disguised. Honesty is the best policy—if I don't treat my disease on a daily basis, I will eventually ingest again, and for me to ingest is to die. Today, I want to live, thank God!

Janice's Jaunt

Quite early—in fourth grade, to be exact—I got moved into a class with kids I didn't know or like very much. My friends, all the really popular ones, were advanced with Mrs. Jones across the hall. I distinctively recall believing that somehow my excessive weight was partly responsible for this humiliating demotion. By fifth grade, toxic thoughts and fears were sadly incorporated into my state of mind, as problems of alcoholism in my home were starting to be apparent.

> *I found that I was subject to huge nightly binges, which would never end when I wanted them to. It didn't deter me when I was actually sick from overeating. Once I ate a snack or two of the very same snacks my family shared, but then they quit! I, on the other hand, binged on, never understanding my strong urges to do so. I reasoned that we just had too much food available to me from our grocery business. But truly, I was baffled as to why I kept eating so much junk food all the time. My weight was interfering with how I thought about myself. But I loved the processed food!*

Processed food is taking an exhilarating part in Janice's life. This was unbeknown to Janice, though, because she was in the hidden stages of the disease of processed food addiction. Notice it is not the cause (processed food) that she discusses; rather, she concentrates on the diagnoses (and there are many in Janice's case) and the symptoms.

> *Then the disease progressed, and I found myself crying over the bed, confused, not knowing what was wrong with me. I could not even follow through when I would swear off junk food just eight hours before. I hated the fact that even though I knew I shouldn't ingest junk food, doing it would always make my disappointments go away, and with this came the illusion that I was going to be okay. Sometimes, when I'd continue to eat, I'd end up feeling high ... a real mood swing. I'd laugh at life then—so what, it didn't matter. After all, everything I wanted to be was happy and thin, which I believed would eventually happen. Bolstered up by ingesting lots of processed food, and having faith, I was sure of it.*
>
> *My family doctor explained my diet choices of meat, starches, white toast, sweets of all forms, and crunchy, salty processed snacks were wrong. So, at fifteen, I was prescribed amphetamines and instructed to "eat an apple" whenever hungry. Ashamed, I didn't explain that my hunger was with me all of the time. So, armed with a doctor's approach to fix me, I determined that if I*

didn't have an appetite, I could stop eating. So, not eating became the goal. I figured since I'd starved all day, a binge, should it ever happen now, could be neutralized. If the food tasted like cardboard, all the better. Then, I wouldn't want it anymore, and then I'd lose the weight that was destroying my happiness.

We can see the either-or thinking here; a person with an active addiction lives in a dichotomous world. Everything is black or white, hot or cold, flat-out or full stop. And here the disease is personified in the dichotomous thinking of "I am either good (right) or I'm bad (wrong)." Janice has labeled her food choices as *wrong*. Taking this a step further, we note the difference between a processed food addict and a non-PFA. As a severe a processed food addict gets older, processed food means more to them. Meanwhile, a non-PFA understands there is a difference between food choices: which are better for them healthwise and which are not. The non-PFA also understands that any food choice, if overeaten, is not conducive to health. Hence, they can moderate, cut down to a more acceptable level, or stop for health reasons. Simply said, the non-PFA has a choice; the processed food addict has lost the power of choice.

I tried smoking first in fifth grade and later used chain smoking as a way to manage the need to eat all the time. I earned a two-and-a-half-pack-a-day habit. I thought doing this plus amphetamines should work.

My teenage friends were all dating. I had the role of best friend to both a girlfriend and her boyfriend. Socially, my weight surely was to blame, so I worked on being perfect, clever, and funny—the things I could control and the things my friends liked about me. I trudged on, very unhappy and wearing a mask of not just being okay but of being really great! The last few years in high school, I overcompensated and compromised by using drugs in the wrong crowd. But after all, it was the 1960s: I could lose all of my issues in that kind of fog.

Note, Janice's addiction is comorbid with other substances.

> *Things were increasingly unmanageable after high school. I was nervous from amphetamines. I was stressed out. I worried about everything and frustrations dominated my thoughts, feelings, and behaviors. On the other hand, I wanted to be happy, and my success and happiness were driven by weight loss. No matter that even on the best of days, the lack of progress with my weight hung over me. I'd eat one cheese sandwich a day and still not lose weight. I figured it must have been the mayonnaise. Also, it was hard to be happy without the food helping my mood. I quit the amphetamines and became very depressed. I tried to vomit after eating, but was unsuccessful. I wanted out of this situation. I was tired, really tired of it. Nothing was working anymore.*

Once again, the processed food addict blames their weight as the problem. I think it is fair to say no one really understood the disease of processed food addiction. Or if there was an understanding, the remedy was a behavioral approach—to fix it. Sure, there are many people who have not crossed the physiological line to addiction, where behavioral methods and other treatment therapies have helped, but with a processed food addict, it is impossible for them to stop through their own willpower. This is no different from the challenge for a real alcoholic.

> *I had to be hospitalized when I was twenty-one years old. After discharge, I did counseling with a therapist and took meditation classes. I developed a more moderate approach to my eating problem, lest I drive myself into the ground and have to go back to the hospital. Then, gladly, I became a born-again Christian. I read somewhere in the Bible that we are not supposed to hate our own flesh. Life then became quite good. I went back to school, got straight A's, met lots of friends, and got married. The food*

issues remained more or less operating in the background. I had resigned to the fact it was there and unfortunately, it is going to be part of me.

"Why not admit and embrace it?" I thought.

People always seemed to identify with losing weight. Because I didn't know how to lose the weight or control my food intake, I now sought to be educated and taught by others on how to control the weight myself. Then came the expensive programs, medications and shots, counseling, counting calories, reconstituting powders, gym memberships, gadgets, videos, hypnosis, self-help books, fads, metabolism experts, only eating proteins, only eating vegetables, studying nutritional charts, low carbs with low fat, and high fat with no carbs.

Drowning in information, I marched on. I also attended, for decades, eating groups that eliminated sugar and wheat, and I identified as being a food addict, but I could not adhere to the food plans long-term. I sooner or later always picked up. I was always baffled as I tried over and over again, putting in the sincerest of efforts each time.

Above are some of the methods Janice has tried with a few more to follow below as the disease continues to progress. It's important to note here, these methods may help others but not a severe processed food addict.

By now in my late thirties, I worked hard in emergency nursing. Breaking both feet after quitting smoking and gaining a hundred-plus pounds, I had to leave my job in ER. After numerous years of desperately trying to lose that much weight, I finally scheduled gastric bypass surgery. This time, I was absolutely sure the nail was going into the coffin. The surgeon strongly warned me that eating sugar would destroy the entire outcome.

I would like to comment on a topic I hear quite often, not only in the clinic but among colleagues who do not understand the disease of processed food addiction. It is quite often said that processed food addiction is nowhere near as bad as alcoholism, drugs, gambling, and so on. I strongly disagree. Many of my patients have lost friends, family, and jobs due to processed food addiction. Not to mention the missed opportunities due to the symptoms of this disease.

Janice point-blank shares she had to leave her job because she was so obese that she fractured her ankles.

I was flying recently for work, and the woman beside me—wait for it—purchased two seats in the plane so she could put the arm rest up and "spread out." My heart went out to her. Whether she is a processed food addict or not is not for me to judge. More importantly, one day I believe that as this disease becomes better known, less stigmatized, *and* understood, individuals will be given some hope that if they are in the mild to moderate stages of processed food addiction (psychologically dependent or at a previous stage), they may be able to do something about it. Prevention is better than remission.

> "Of course," I assured him, "I don't like sugar, doctor. My problem is with pastas and corn chips."
>
> Like whistling in the dark, I thought I could at least manage eliminating sugar from my diet, and I sincerely meant it. It was a hard process, but I got through the surgery. Too bad that every time the bariatric support groups met, I had a scheduled shift and never attended one of those meetings, although deep down inside I knew something was different about me. So, I continued to work on my sugar and flour intake myself.
>
> The next five years were weird. Sweets were more of a problem than I was apparently aware of. If I pushed to eat more, I'd get sick and vomit. My ideas about food and how to control it were still operating. My final bariatric outcome was far from stellar,

falling short by 70 lb. of what had been decided as a reasonable goal weight for me. But at least I could maintain an 80 lb. loss, I hoped. After all, I was "fixed."

The processed food addict is always hoping against hope that somehow, someway, someday they will *control* (see below) and enjoy their ingestion of processed food.

Then, while working as a supervisor in an outpatient setting, I got the notion that I should make my patients' lives more fun—to give back in a way, and to be a blessing to others. So, I started hosting big parties for everyone on the unit, all at my expense. Typically, we'd have eight extra-large pizzas, 125 chicken wings, six 2-liter sodas, various sides of french fries, potato salads, and slaws, all delivered. Then, I would go out to get dessert for thirty-five people. I would spend a lot of time on what to order, when to order, and how much to order. Although it was expensive, usually around $250 each time, I kept ordering up with these parties over and over again. I would stand there and watch everyone eat and, mostly, I would not eat. It would feel to me that I now had some control.

Another weird thing was that my staff kept bragging about their great success at a casino in West Virginia. I had played some slots before, but there didn't seem much point to it. I just went there to see what they were talking about, taking my eighty-five-year-old father along. We both won about a hundred dollars each. My dad had fun, but I immediately deduced that gambling would become an easy and profitable part-time job. Smitten with the belief that I possessed a skill to read machines, that very night I launched into a sixteen-year compulsive gambling addiction. Gambling, its excitement, and the action sort of replaced an experience I had been missing. Magically, I didn't even think of processed food while betting away the hours. But whenever I attempted to quit gambling, the processed food ingestion would exacerbate. And every new diet cycle brought on more cravings to gamble.

They call it "switching the witch for the bitch."

Progressively, I could not keep my own personal finances straight. Once very competent with money, I could not keep an ATM card—even though our savings account remained pretty much at zero. Good thing was I didn't need gambling to live like I did with processed food.

Then, in the late summer of 2016, with my weight alarmingly heading very north again, I realized that I needed real professional help in some way with this junk-food addiction. A friend invited me to a workshop presented by Dr. Karren-Lee Raymond, who was visiting Baltimore, Maryland. Her insight and knowledge of my regretful, merciless condition was so profound it was astonishing—the fact that my brain and body will react differently, not just to sugar and wheat, which I was led to believe was the case, but to all processed foods, was astounding. Just like other people with diseases, I too had a recognized chronic disease, similar to alcoholism, defined as processed food addiction.

What's more, I learned my disease could be sparked off by eating non-processed food, telling myself at least I wouldn't put on as much weight and that I was being good, as it was healthy food. Little did I know it was only a matter of time before my rationalizing head would say, "You can control non-processed food now, so one cookie won't hurt." I would sooner or later be off to the races again, ingesting all that was in sight.

I further learned Dr. Raymond had been treating other patients effectively and successfully. I learned that it wasn't my fault, it wasn't psychological or because of my parents or a dysfunctional childhood, and more importantly, I could actually recover from it.

Wow! My disease of processed food addiction would remain in remission forever, as long as I treated it daily.

The lights became glaringly bright upon hearing these initial truths (there have been many others over the past two-plus-years). It caused within me a psychic shift. By fall of 2016, I was working on living in the solution with her. Within a time frame of sixty-plus years and failing at my own best efforts, I realize that God had done for me what I couldn't do for myself. The problem is simply lifted. My mind is clear, and my body is exactly where it should be (albeit over a hundred pounds lighter). In liberation, I learned that obesity and weight are just symptoms of my problem—processed food addiction—and not the cause of my many pressing issues. I live life today as it comes to me. I now am finally free.

Shandell Shares

I started eating processed food very young in life. I remember sneaking into the kitchen at a very early age of around four or five, taking cookies from the cookie jar, and sneaking back to my bed when my parents had just gone off to sleep. The following night, I did the exact same thing; however, I took more cookies. I used to get upset when there were no cream-filled cookies left so I had to have the plain or chocolate chip instead. This always upset me, as I preferred the cream cookies.

Many children in their early years of life have been exposed to processed foods, making them vulnerable to addiction later. Will this be the case for Shandell?

I loved it when my Nan baked cakes. I was the first one to help out, as she would let us lick the beaters and the bowl afterwards. Whether it was licking the cake batter or licking the icing on the beaters, it didn't matter. I loved it all—I remember thinking how yummy they were and didn't want my licking to come to an end.

> *I picked up cigarettes at an early age, too, then alcohol, and on to recreational drugs. However, I know today that processed food is my first drug of choice—my primary addiction. Nothing felt quite as good as taking that first bite of the processed food I was about to devour.*

Once again, multi-comorbidity appears among a smorgasbord (pardon the pun) of substances.

> *Pain was my greatest persuader; I knew that I wasn't well and needed help. I attended an OA meeting and didn't really like or understand what they were sharing, but I can see now I didn't identify with them. I couldn't moderate my meals—one was too many and a hundred bites of processed food were not enough! I then came across FA (Food Addiction in Recovery). I lasted eighteen months in that fellowship, and that was where I first got abstinent. I then progressed into FAA (Food Addicts Anonymous), which I only hung around for a short period. I couldn't seem to keep my abstinence, which pushed me into RFA (Recovery from Food Addiction). I was in that fellowship for about a year or so and had seven months of abstinence up. But then, once again, the mental twist kicked in—out of the blue, and before I knew it, I was off again. My life was consumed by dieting, restricting, purging, slogging out at the gym, fun runs, constantly on and off the scales, weight-loss centers, professionals, organic food only, in and out of self-help groups of all letters and acronyms, and the list goes on ...*

> *Even though I learned a lot from the various self-help groups, my head noise chatter was driving me insane. I felt like a dry drunk, which I came to know as an empty processed food addict. Deep down inside of me, I wanted to be normal, or be able to control my processed food intake just like I saw others doing who shared they were in recovery. I couldn't for the life of me understand how some people could eat a little bit extra or even overingest on non-processed*

foods AND get away with it. My head would go off—I would feel guilty, remorseful, fat, a failure once again, especially as I saw others being able to do this with some normalcy but I couldn't. I still wanted the processed food—it was like when I didn't ingest it, I felt crap, and when I did ingest it, I felt even worse. I was doomed if I did and doomed if I didn't. But I was desperate to find some sort of recovery that would help my head shut up and my processed food intake stop with some sort of quietness in my mind.

So, I sought help on July 4, 2016. This help came from an addictionologist (with a PhD in psychology and specifically in processed food addiction). Once I learned and understood (in my heart of hearts) about the disease of addiction and accepted that I was a processed food addict, I finally got some peace—peace from my disease, my illness, that had been always telling me how bad, unworthy, lazy, ungrateful, not good enough, not perfect enough I was ... peace that I was not fighting the diagnosis any more; the list is endless. I came to understand I was not my disease, similar to a person who has, for example, type 2 diabetes. The diabetes does not define who that person is.

It was like I was waking up out of a coma—starting to see things in a different light. Dr. Raymond helped me to understand my disease of processed food addiction and, more importantly, offered me hope with a solution, guiding me to make contacts with others who have also recovered from this seemingly futile way of living in which it seemed there was no point to life.

Today, I treat my disease by eliminating all processed food while weighing my portions, which provides me with enough energy to live my life on a daily basis. My weight has stabilized within 5 lb. (2 kg.) every month—some months I might be up a couple of pounds or so and other months I might be down a couple of pounds or so, but the majority of the time I am around the same number on the scale. More importantly, that number on the scale, my weight, *doesn't define who I am today. Admittedly, I have come to understand I am human and sometimes, for example, if it is that time of the month and I feel a bit bloated, my odap (my dickhead addiction personality named tish—mixture of sh_ _) may whisper a sweet nothing in my ear. I know that this is NOT due to me bingeing on processed foods and not anything to do with my old active life in the disease, but that this is normal today. There is so much freedom in knowing AND understanding this.*

Even more so, having the disease of processed food addiction does not define who I am today. I am learning I am so much more. I also attend a 12 step meeting where I meet other recovered processed food addicts. Together, we learn how to continually live a spiritual way of life—helping each other to stay honest about ourselves each day and what is happening in that big world out there. We share regularly on the phone and face-to-face and are always ready to help each other if and whenever we can. We meet regularly all around the world, this being one of the highlights of recovery. I look forward to it, the love, the laughter, the encouragement of each other, the empathy shown to someone who is where I used to be. Weight was only a symptom. There is no competition of who has been abstinent the longest, or lost the most weight, or sponsors the most people. I don't have to do anything. Just treat my disease on a daily basis. That is, I do not ingest processed foods or any other substance to cope with life today. I am learning how to live life on life's terms.

I went to bed last night as a processed food addict and woke up this morning as a processed food addict—this is honesty for me at its core. I am so blessed to have found the solution and I'm very grateful for my new life. And they tell me it keeps getting better.

Here's an update on where I am today, a couple more years down the track. So, having worked with Dr. Raymond, my life has certainly turned around for the better. Her personal touch, along with professional expertise in addiction (specifically, processed food addiction), has enabled me to study, change careers, and get work in a field that I had only dreamed of doing, let alone actually achieving it.

As well as getting my health back, finding clarity in my decision-making, and gaining a positive outlook on life, I never thought I would ever be able to be living a life I have today, and the noise in my head has finally subsided! AND ... I only see my addictionologist now if and when I need to. I liken it to, if I have a sore tooth, I see my dentist; if something is threatening my recovery from this disease, I know I am not alone today, primarily with my recovery buddies, plus a specialist who I know I can get in touch with at any time.

The effectiveness of my practice in treating addiction, specifically processed food addiction, is founded on the premise of "I aspire to do myself out of a job." This means, from the time I first diagnose and treat a patient who has the disease of addiction, my intention is always for the disease to go into remission. For example, a cancer may not grow or spread if the patient is treated. The addiction will still be in remission. Hence, treating their disease on a daily basis helps the individual's disease stay in complete remission. Even though the cancer is still present, it does not go away and stay away—it's not cured. More importantly, the patient post-treatment is encouraged to learn how to live in society while continuing to treat their disease. There are millions of people globally who can attest their disease of addiction is in remission and who continue to actively work toward *living life to the fullest.*

As a professional working in the addiction arena, I actively continue to seek bio-psycho-social-spiritual professional instruction in the treatment of addiction. I believe this is essential in such a specialized field of counseling and treatment. This allows me to play a central role in transforming the health of the patient. The ultimate objective of any health-care specialist is to improve the patient's health and medical care, so that the person may feel herself part of society as a whole, and know that society voluntarily accepts her as she is.

Of course, I have patients who decide this is not for them, or want to do things another way, or relapse and decide this is not for them. At the very least, I believe the person has learned something about the disease of processed food addiction, and if in the future they are a processed food addict, they know they are not alone and help is available.

Betty's Bio

Betty's story is a testament to age not being a barrier to recovery. Whether younger or older, it does not matter. Blessedly, Betty's disease was able to be treated, giving her a new outlook on life, which is not blurred by the processed food addiction any longer.

> *Hi, my name is Betty. I am a little older than most people I know who have recovered from the disease of processed food addiction. I also have learned that this disease doesn't distinguish between race, creed, color, age, sex, or vocation. I survived!*
>
> *I grew up on a dairy farm in Maryland. I had a younger brother. My dad was a hard worker and one of thirteen children. My mother was the youngest of seven children—only three lived to adulthood. There is a lot of hard work on a dairy farm. My mother had to fill in at times. As we got older, my brother was to help out on the farm, but I was a girl, so I had to do the work inside the house.*
>
> *On the farm, I felt lonely, isolated, and fearful. My brother, four years younger than me, could work in the fields, and although my mother sometimes worked in the fields, I wasn't allowed to. My chores were to do things like the dishes or other housework. So, I thought I wasn't good enough to do the "fun things." My mother thought she was protecting me.*

With Betty, we can see once again that weight is one of (if not *the*) the major symptoms of processed food addiction, being the most important thing for every processed food addict. Importantly, one does not have to be overweight or underweight. The overweight individuals try their hardest to get the weight off; the underweight try their darnedest to keep the weight down, and down and down. The more weight a person loses, the more euphoric they feel, the more in control they feel; once again, this is evidence that they can't possibly be a processed food addict.

> *I am not sure when I first knew I was overweight, but I believe it was around the age of five. I remember asking Santa for a cowgirl outfit at about that age. I got it, but it was too small. I was very disappointed. My mother seemed disappointed. My entire family—my parents, my brother, my grandparents (on both sides of the family), and aunts and uncles—were overweight.*
>
> *One experience I remember was, I think, probably in second grade. We went across the street to the playground to eat our lunch. My lunch box wasn't closed properly, and my lunch fell out. One of my classmates thought it was very funny. I am not sure if I was more upset about him laughing or about losing my lunch. It was terribly embarrassing, and I felt very hurt.*
>
> *I started school at five and a half. I was shy and scared. I have no memory of being told that I would be going to school or what to expect. I remember asking one of the girls to be my friend. She agreed but seemed annoyed, saying "I can't do everything for you."*
>
> *When my mother took me to the doctor, he made a comment about my weight. She seemed embarrassed, and there was some attempt to cut down on ingesting sweets, but it seemed impossible. If my parents were out some place and saw people they hadn't seen for a while, the friend would comment about how "healthy" my brother and I were. I know the word* healthy *has a different meaning today*

than when I was growing up. Even though they made no mention about my weight, I knew on some level it was about my weight.

Once in my mid-teens, my mother and I tried to lose weight without success. I married at twenty and had two sons. After a few months, we moved to a small house on the farm. My husband and I separated when my second son was three weeks old. Very soon after that, I got a job in order to support myself and my sons. I continued to live on the farm, but by the time my oldest son was in kindergarten, I found a place near my job, so we moved from the farm.

My mother didn't think I should date. I was then the mother of two sons, working, raising them, and going to college to get a better job. Again, I was different than the people around me. I found it too hard to participate in after-school activities like my fellow students. I was always struggling with my weight and felt less than other people, thinking they didn't want to be around me.

Some of my recollection is that I started in Overeaters Anonymous in the early seventies. I was in my fifties, I think. I went to meetings, stayed to the end, got up, and left the meeting without asking anyone to help me, be my sponsor, or try to learn more about the program. For years, I was in and out of OA while looking for other programs to lose weight, which I did several of to no avail, as I would lose weight only to gain it back again. One program had liquid protein that I drank, ingesting no solid food. I lost weight, but as always, I would put it right back on again, and even more when I quit the program.

I found out about a treatment center in Arizona that treated eating disorders, alcoholics, codependents, and sex addicts. I went to Arizona for one month of treatment. It cost quite a lot in those days, but I needed and wanted help. I couldn't understand why some people in OA and other diet groups were doing fine and I wasn't. It too worked for a while, BUT ... I was off again, regaining my weight and some more as well.

I started attending workshops two or three times a year. Some were up to three days. Others were longer workshops on food addiction, relapse preventions, healing my brain, learning how to deal with resentment, with forgiveness, and more. But the whole time my weight kept going up and down—nothing was changing!!! As I started each of the programs, I felt hopeful this would be "the one." Sometimes, it lasted for a few months, but eventually I was not able to maintain abstinence or stick to the food plan of the time. I journaled and sometimes jotted down my weight. A few years ago, I totaled all the information and it added up to be over one thousand pounds!!!

I guess I was hopeless back then, now that I look at it, but I didn't know I was suffering from a disease of addiction—processed food addiction. I could be abstinent for short periods of time but always went back to the processed food. I was discouraged, scared, and angry.

Here I was, seventy-eight years old, and still had no control over my intake of processed food—I especially loved the sweet treats but would binge on anything that was in the cupboard or was at my local church group. Or I would start at someplace and then come home and "go for it," saying, "What's the use, anyhow? I might as well make the most of it."

Sometimes, I didn't think at all! My weight kept going up and down. There were so many temptations and people insisting I have one little bite. If I had one bite, I might not stop for weeks, months, or years. The worst part for me was the morning after the binge. My odap, which I name S_ _ _ head, would start: "You've done it again; no one will like you; you are weak and pathetic; it is all your fault; you have just gained 20 lb." The rhetorical voice ... the messages went on and on. Most people never understood, especially some of our international friends.

I was balancing work, school, and raising two sons. On and off food programs with some success, but inevitably these always led to failure, but I was always hoping that I would learn to control my food intake. There was always one more attempt AND one more failure. But some of those around me seemed to be succeeding. "What was wrong with me?" I wondered.

In 1975, I got married again to a kind man who has been loving and supportive over the years, even with my weight gains and losses. He had three children who came to live with us. At that time, they were nine, eleven, and thirteen. He took over seeing that we all ate. He loved all kinds of pasta, ice cream, and so on. So, here I was again, facing lots of yummy foods. My husband loves to cook, but they are meals that I do not ingest today, or they will spark off my allergy—a phenomenon of craving that I have come to understand—so, for me, I CANNOT EAT those foods or if I do, I will suffer dire consequences. I have had a psychic change, and I know the difference today.

About two years ago, I learned that a friend I knew from a 12 step food program who had been struggling like me was having success with weight loss.

She was working with an addictionologist from Australia. Then three other friends who I knew from one of my last 12 step food groups also seemed to have success—not only in weight loss, but they seemed so much happier, and said the obsession had been removed, and more importantly to them, the voice had quieted right down. So, at age seventy-eight, I started working with Dr. Raymond, or should I say K-L, which is how I came to know her.

At first, it wasn't easy. I had to let go of ALL my old ideas about weight, food, control, and fear, and that, at first, was challenging, as I liked to be in control. But as K-L shared, "See where 'me in charge' got me thus far!"

My whole life had been about how to get rid of my weight and keep it off, while continually trying to learn how to eat what I wanted, when I wanted, how I wanted, and where I wanted. Plus enjoy it too!

Today, I can say my recovery journey has been so worth it.

I started working with Dr. Raymond, who helped me to understand my disease. She often said to me, "Self-knowledge will avail you nothing, Betty. You can know and learn everything you can about weight, dieting, self-help books, and food plans, but it isn't going to make you a normal eater."

I liked it when she shared so simply to me. It made sense for the first time. This "thing" I had was not my fault. She talked about how the same goes for others with a chronic disease and gave me the example of someone who has a chronic illness such as a person with diabetes. They can learn everything there is to know about diabetes, but they still can't fix their pancreas no matter what knowledge they have.

She also shared with me that this disease is the only disease to her knowledge that tells the individual they don't have a disease. I could so relate to that, too. I could go to bed in the early days of treatment and recovery knowing I was a processed food addict, but come morning, I would forget again.

Today, recovery is about learning and understanding I have a disease—an addiction—that can't be fixed but can be treated, one day at a time. Hence today, I now treat my disease.

You see, for so many years, I knew I had a problem. Anyone could see that, but I never had a solution. My solution was always to lose weight, and so I would do anything and everything for that to happen. While I was busy doing that over many decades, my disease of processed food addiction eluded me. I didn't want to be a processed food addict, so part of the denial was me trying to be normal or to call it by another label—compulsive overeater, emotional eater, food addict. I think it is only now that someone has come up with a solution that I can accept it. That someone who offered the solution relied a lot on her own personal experience—not only knowing about my disease professionally but also having lived it herself and recovered.

I learned it was impossible for a food addict to eliminate food. That was like a drink addict trying to give up drinking. Slowly, things started to make sense and I came to understand I had been suffering from a disease, and it had a name—processed food addiction. K-L helped me understand that I had a mental obsession and a physical allergy that no amount of willpower could overcome. The only remedy she has come to know is entire abstinence for a real processed food addict.

So, here I am, now eighty years old, and I have a very different way of life that I never thought was possible. I now know how to treat my disease on a daily basis—and for the first time I have success in weight loss: it just hasn't come back on. As K-L shares with me, "Weight and everything that goes with it are symptoms of the underlying cause—processed food addiction—just like being drunk or wobbling down the street are symptoms of the underlying cause, alcoholism."

Of course, that made sense; if I don't ingest processed foods then I won't put on weight or be obsessed with weight like I had been imprisoned for so many years. I guess if an alcoholic doesn't drink alcohol, they won't get drunk.

Today, I continue to work to remain free from the shackles of weight, dieting, fear, shame, guilt, and anxiety. I learned that it is not about staying on my food plan—I couldn't do that in a million years and I have lots of proof of that too. It is about coming to first understand I have an illness, a disease of addiction AND being treated by someone who understands and has the professional and academic knowledge needed to treat addiction. Then taking steps to eliminate all the processed food and then learning how to live without it. I can make better choices and do not binge today. I cook all my food and look forward to meals, knowing that I am eating a healthy, abstinent,

> *clean meal. I attend a 12 step fellowship on a Tuesday night and we go out to dinner at a local restaurant after my meeting. I feel good, physically and emotionally. I continue to learn more about the spiritual side of things as I continue to grow and get more honest with myself. I was a professional in my field of social work, and through recovery, I now hold two women's meetings a month, where more mature women come and sit down in my home and we just all talk and share together. I feel useful today.*
>
> *I am so, so grateful to Karren-Lee. First of all, she gave me hope, and then she treated me and taught me how to get free from the shackles of weight, dieting, fear, shame, guilt, and anxiety. But most importantly, I have been relieved of the fears of putting on weight again—so long as I continue to treat my disease on a daily basis, while continuing to establish a relationship with this higher power that I am only coming to understand and know as God—LOVE.*

Karen's Case

Once again, in the preliminary stages, we don't know if a person is a processed food addict or not. Taking another look at the paradigm of the phases of processed food addiction, many babies are exposed to processed foods. If we take this a step further, and there is a genetic predisposition to be a potential processed food addict, then a baby maybe vulnerable to this disease.

> *When I was a baby, I always cried for more milk. My mother said I was the only one that never got enough. As a toddler, I remember always feeling bigger than the others. I felt so embarrassed about my weight even at such a young age. I was always supersensitive, crying at the slightest criticisms of me. If someone looked at me the wrong way, or raised their voice at me, I just cried, and I didn't know why. I got teased as an overweight kid and it got worse when I attended junior high school and the kids were mean. Today, it*

> would be labeled bullying. I always ate more than my friends. I couldn't understand how they could stop when they were full, as I always felt compelled to have more.

It is important to note in Karen's case her sharing about being supersensitive. Addiction and the personality trait of being emotionally sensitive go hand in hand. Addicts by nature are known to be highly sensitive, although many research articles concur that approximately 15 to 20 percent of society have a highly sensitive nature. Whether it is an innate trait or a characteristic that comes with the territory of addiction, I do not know. Clinically, though, I can attest that my patients are sensitive individuals with a tendency to perfectionism. It appears to take an extended period of time for the person with addiction to acquire the maturity needed to outgrow such an acute affliction.

> I started attending diet workshops and Weight Watchers with my mom, to no avail. Now I think about it, there were innumerable diets that I tried, including Atkins, all-shake diet, Jenny Craig, Nutri System, all-salad diet, fen-phen (which I found out was fatal for some people). Getting on the scale every week was so embarrassing. "You only lost a quarter of a pound" and "This week you gained half a pound."

> My life began to be dictated by the number on that scale. Then my whole family went on a diet, and I was the one who stayed on it the longest—I felt so proud of myself. But it wasn't long before I gained the weight and then some. Senior high was much the same, only my weight continued to increase, and my self-esteem plummeted. At college, I gained more than the "freshman 15"; it was more like the "freshman 30."

> I finally graduated and then entered the workforce. I remember my sister getting married and I didn't want to be left behind a spinster. I knew I had to lose weight to find my future husband,

so I starved myself. I got down to 135 lb. and found my man. After I got engaged, my weight started to climb higher than ever, as we frequented more and more restaurants and ate takeout all the time. I found I couldn't control the amount of food I was eating no matter how hard I tried.

I would order takeout pizza, cheesesteak subs, fries, and a Coke. I promised myself I would only eat two slices of pizza and leave the sub and fries for my husband, but I ended up eating all the pizza, half the sub, and the fries before I even got home.

This continued, BUT then it was time to start my next diet to end all diets, as I was getting married. Hallelujah, I lost 20 lb., but I didn't lose the 50 lb. that was my goal from the onset. Then I got pregnant with my first child and gained 50 lb.—I couldn't stop eating sugar, sugar, sugar and processed foods in all forms. This weight stayed on.

Then I swore that for my second pregnancy, I wasn't going to gain any more weight, but I still gained a further 18 lb. Yes, I was morbidly overweight, much to my embarrassment, especially when all the women in my husband's family were super thin and health-conscious. His mother was very worried about my weight, as she knew my father was very obese and I was on my way to being just like him. She was on my case even more than my own mother; therefore, my husband started to get on my case. This was very humiliating.

Karen's story also touches on the role of genetics in processed food addiction. Ongoing research continues to support a physical foundation for alcoholism; that is, those individuals who are genetically predisposed to alcoholism have a higher risk of developing alcoholism. In fact, the child of one parent with alcoholism has approximately a twenty-five percent chance of developing alcoholism. If both parents are alcoholics, the chances of the child being alcoholic are doubled. We can see in these case studies that processed food addiction began in the very early years of the individual. In the oncoming years, I believe processed food will go down a similar path—exposing it to also having a genetic predisposition.

> *I then had the kids, and still tried to control my eating but still to no avail, as I was eating what they were eating—plus all their leftover foods.*
>
> *Next, I heard about a 12 step food program, which I started to attend. I got some hope in the beginning when I started to lose some weight, but again, that didn't last for more than three months. I tried and tried to be like the others, who seemed to be abstinent and getting away with some extra food on the side. I tried everything I could to be like them, but I always ended up overeating on non-processed food, which always sooner or later led me to the processed foods. I questioned myself endlessly: what was wrong with me? I cried in the meetings because I just couldn't seem to get it. This lasted for a whole thirteen years.*
>
> *Then I started praying for someone to help me with the steps, but after eight sponsors, who all fired me for not staying abstinent, things were going downhill pretty fast. Then I was connected to a person who treated processed food addiction, although I did not know that at the time. To be honest, I did know such a person existed. She needed a ride and, in the car, I told her my woes, that they couldn't help me with the steps. I had done the steps many times but always busted. I have since learned the 12 step program could not help me because I didn't understand I had a disease known as processed food addiction This was the first step toward the freedom and liberation I have today.*

I have been noticing lately a lot more relapses, empty processed food addicts, and substance abusers who have eliminated the substances but nothing else has changed. They are staying this way due to self-knowledge, as well as attending seven-plus meetings a week of a 12 step fellowship and making multiple calls to stay off the substance. If it works for the person, they are happy, and their life is manageable, then it is none of my business. However, I believe as we move more and more into the twenty-first century, processed food addiction is heading into the scientific field of promoting solutions while the patient is still trying to come to terms that they may have a disease.

> I was asked to do service and pick up Dr. Karren-Lee Raymond from the airport. I did not know who I was picking up, but I knew she was important—she does not like to be seen like that, as I was to find out later on. Neither Dr. Raymond nor I were given each other's contact information, so we could not find each other. After several hours circling the airport to find her, and just as I was about to give up, we found one another.
>
> We had missed the retreat, but both of us had our dinner loaves, so we ate them as we got to know one another. We then stayed up until 3:00 a.m. the next morning, as she was teaching me about the disease of addiction. I finally had some hope, and for the first time started to see I had a disease, that I wasn't weak-willed, a glutton, or the worst person in the world, but that I had a chronic illness known as processed food addiction, PFA. It felt as though a ton of bricks was being lifted off my shoulders.
>
> Then I got into professional treatment for my addiction. This proved to be my saving grace. Just like someone else with a chronic illness, such as diabetes, cardiac disease, or cancer, before the treatment can be implemented effectively, the patient must know and understand what is going on with them. That was another thing I had to come to terms with: me being a patient. That meant I was sick. Not crazy, just sick. Dr. Raymond shared that in the early days of recovery I would be convalescing—treating my disease. I couldn't understand something if I didn't know what it was. This

was the beginning of the end for me. I heard there was a solution to a problem I now could begin to understand.

What transpired was Dr. Raymond treated me for the disease of processed food addiction—the key word here is addiction. *I can see, and now understand, I am just like an alcoholic—they eliminate alcohol, I eliminate processed foods. Part of Dr. Raymond's treatment was for me to attend a 12 step self-help group while I worked with her. I learned that my processed food addiction was the tip of the iceberg, and once it was in remission, we then worked on what underpinned my disease of processed food addiction. I could then start to learn how to live in the world out there without a substance.*

Every day is a miracle. I have been reunited with my sons, my family, and my coworkers. I have taken on advanced education classes, faced some financial upheavals, and had relationship challenges and I have stayed abstinent, sober, and clean, with peace of mind. I am so grateful to have been given the solution and treatment guidelines to my fatal malady—I'm not alone today.

"Together, we can."

Afterword

The words throughout this book highlight an innovative area of addiction, especially in the twenty-first century, where there continues to be an upsurge in the consequences of this chronic illness.

Am I a processed food addict?

This is a question I confidently assume will be spoken about, written about, investigated, and debated to a state of prolonged public dispute—or, if you like, a point of controversy—among many non-processed food addicts and potential processed food addicts, in academia, medicine, religion, and (let's not forget) our writers and editors in the print media and society's ever-growing social media. That being said, I feel obliged to share briefly, or more aptly, personally encapsulate a few last words, *food for thought* ...

I have been asked many times over the past decade to write a book about processed food addiction being an illness. What I have written in the previous chapters is not a universal panacea, nor a magic antidote. It was written to simply inform non-professionals in the field of addiction—the person who may identify with some of the cases in this book, or the individual who has a relative, friend, colleague, or perhaps a brother, sister, mother, or father who is constantly battling weight, body image, processed food consumption, or even life. Additionally, I hope our professional friends in addiction medicine, the health domains, and ministries of all denominations may find useful information here.

I know only too well what it is like standing in the firing line. I witness the tragedies and the desperation of family members (to say the least) and all those in the wake of the disease of addiction, a destructive and merciless malady. It is gut-wrenching and heartbreaking to contemplate that, at this very moment, someone somewhere in the world has just binged their way through a mountain of processed food, vomited their little heart out, gulped down twenty-plus laxatives, run five miles (8 k.), or just gotten off the scales wanting to die because they saw 275 lb. (125 kg.) or more, or at the other end of the scale, 90 lb. (40 kg.).

In the background, they are taunted and teased by the disease voice, saying, "You have done it again" or "You are still not thin enough" or "You are a pathetic excuse for a human being." Yes, the aftereffects are self-punishment, anger, hopelessness, heightened fear of uncertainty, and bewilderment, and the list goes on.

It is also important to consider parents, spouses, family, friends, colleagues, professionals, and non-professionals who so desperately pray and hope that one day, somehow, their loved one will wake up and be free of this merciless disease. At the end of the day, I know I too am human and can only do so much. That is why this book is so important.

Yes, some of your questions will have been answered by what you have read. However, this disease of *processed food addiction*, which is becoming more present in today's society, is far too complex to be treated conclusively in a single piece of literature. In fact, that is a large part of the dilemma we are facing, and the primary reason I have tried to break through the infinite myths, uncertainty, and misconceptions in society on the topic of problems and secondary complications associated with processed food.

More importantly, I want this book to be taken at face value for what it is—not a social, psychological, scientific commentary, but an encouraging treatise. Hence, it is *my sincere hope* that this piece of literature will, as a beacon, give a growing light of hope to all those suffering from the devastating consequences of this chronic disease. This is a disease many men and women—both professional and non-professional—know very little about. Many scoff at it, due to ignorance, as they have little understanding of this disease (for now).

I had a patient only last month who had applied for a scholarship to attend a conference to help her with her addiction. As she was *only* a processed food addict, she was told that her disease was not bad enough or life-threatening enough to warrant a scholarship. Paradoxically, this patient is a professional, her practice is nearly bankrupt, she owes thousands of dollars to the IRS, she drives a car that is only just road-worthy, her family is estranged, her husband has left, and her children are not talking to her. In addition, she is suffering many medical complications, including type 2 diabetes, hypertension, and stress. Need I go on? Her waking hours are dictated by her disease of processed food addiction. In between clients, she is bingeing on graham crackers with peanut butter, candy, and coffee with creamer, just so she can function for the next patient. This is what I mean when I say my heart breaks.

I hope you have found a hope that has eluded so many suffering individuals (who are growing in numbers) for far too long, a hope of release from processed food addiction's devastating grip, and that you too may "arise, and take up your bed and walk"—walk free—free from the disease of processed food addiction.

> *Not that he wishes and prays for does a man get, but what he justly earns. His wishes and prayers are only gratified and answered when they harmonize with his thoughts and actions. In the light of this truth, what, then is the meaning of "fighting against circumstances"? It means that a man is continually revolting against an effect without, while all the time he is nourishing and preserving its cause in his heart. That cause may take the form of a conscious vice or an unconscious weakness; but whatever it is, it*

stubbornly retards the efforts of its possessor, and this calls aloud for a remedy.

(James Allen, As a Man Thinketh)

Appendix A

12-Step Self-Help Groups

Self-help 12-step fellowships for addicts and for the loved ones, families, friends, and colleagues of addicts include the following:

Al-Anon and Alateen

Alcoholics Anonymous (AA): www.aa.org

Compulsive Eaters Anonymous–Honesty, Open-Mindedness, Willingness (CEA-HOW)

Food Addicts Anonymous (FAA)

Nar-Anon and Narateen

Narcotics Anonymous (NA): www.na.org

Overeaters Anonymous (OA)

Processed Food Anonymous (PFA): processedfoodanonymous.org

Processed Food-Anon

Recovery from Food Addiction Anonymous (RFA)

Appendix B

CDs, DVDs, Literature, Services, and Products in the Broad Field of Addiction

Here are just a few examples to begin with.

The AA website has a selection of videos, audios and literature: www.aa.org

Hazelden Publishing: www.hazelden.org/web/public/publishing.page

Dicobe Media Inc.: www.dicobe.com

email: dicobesales@dicobe.com

Appendix C

Country Help Lines

Please call your country help line if in crisis.

Australia

Lifeline Australia—13 11 14. Crisis Support and Suicide Prevention

Canada

Canada Suicide Prevention Service (CSPS), by Crisis Services Canada, enables callers anywhere in Canada to access crisis support using the technology of their choice (phone, text, or chat), in French and English. Phone: toll-free 1-833-456-4566, available 24-7. Text: 45645, available 5:00 p.m.–1:00 a.m. ET. Chat: crisisservicescanada.ca, available 5:00 p.m.–1:00 a.m. ET

UK

Volunteer for Crisis. 66 Commercial Street, London, E1 6LT. Tel: 0300 636 1967 Registered Charity Numbers: E&W1082947, SC040094. http://www.crisis.org.uk

USA

National Suicide Prevention Lifeline: 1-800-273-TALK (8255)
Crisis Text Line (all ages, 24-7): text MATTERS to 741741
Lifeline Crisis Chat: www.contact-usa.org/chat.html
LGBT National Hotline: 1-888-843-4564

Glossary

A1c test (also known as HbA1c): The A1c test is a blood test that evaluates and provides information about a person's average amount of glucose in the blood over the last two to three months. The A1c test is utilized to diagnose prediabetes and type 2 diabetes.

Abstinence: In the preliminary stage of abstinence, the individual eliminates all processed food. However, this alone cannot keep a processed food addict's disease in remission long-term. The foundation of permanent abstinence from processed food addiction is coming to understand their disease both subliminally and consciously. This is stage two, in which a change of heart takes place in the individual as they come to understand the nature of their disease:

how it developed;

how it has affected them neurologically;

how it brings about significant changes in personality, actions and attitudes;

why ingesting processed food makes them feel better;

why the desire to ingest can still occur randomly, especially in the early stages of recovery;

why they cannot safely ingest processed foods; and most importantly, why they will relapse if the disease is not treated.

At the third stage, an inner knowing takes place, leading to permanent abstinence, in which they move beyond the processed food addiction to living a fuller life. This (abstinence) is an adjustment period of living in the world without a substance—that is, learning a new lifestyle—a life without processed food, while they learn to face life on life's terms successfully. The processed food addict eventually experiences peace of mind, having been released from the addiction and its consequences, ultimately moving beyond the processed food addiction; seeking continual balance in the biological, psychological, social, and spiritual aspects of health and well-being.

Addiction: The term *addiction* has been and continues to be debated to this day among professionals and non-professionals. For a processed food addict, *addiction* is defined as a chronic disease with many secondary complications that are the consequence (whether harmful or not) of an apparently innate inability to moderate or stop ingesting processed food. The processed food addict is enslaved, fixated, and dependent on proving they can ingest processed foods like normal people. Addiction is primarily a disease of denial—the only disease I know that tells the patient they don't have a disease and this time it will be different. Once the processed food addict picks up again due to the mental obsession (mental twist), this in turn sparks of a physical craving (physical allergy) which enforces the addict to keep on ingesting, continually destroying the mind. The processed food addict cannot quit ingesting processed food because of the body (physical allergy) and cannot quit because of the mental twist that exists in the mind. Hence the processed food addict is powerless over processed food and their life is certainly going to become unmanageable sooner or later.

Addiction medicine: A medical specialty that is concerned with the prevention, evaluation, diagnosis, treatment, and recovery of individuals with the disease of addiction. This specialty may also deal with family members whose lives are unmanageable due to the impact of a loved one's substance use or addiction.

Addictionist: An addiction specialist. A medical doctor additionally certified by the American Society of Addiction Medicine (ASAM) or the American Board of Addiction Medicine (ABAM).

Addictionologist: Addiction plus psychology brings the professional title of addictionologist. I am a practitioner with a PhD in psychology; my doctorate was specifically in processed food addiction. I have had scientific and academic instruction in the field of addiction medicine, which is essential in such specialized treatment and therapy.

Anhedonia: Loss of the capacity to experience pleasure or gain the pleasures that are ordinarily desirable or appealing. Anhedonia is a typical clinical feature of many health conditions and is frequently associated with addiction, especially during acute withdrawal.

Attention deficit hyperactivity disorder (ADHD): A term used to describe patterns of behavior, which are present in various settings including home and school. It can result in performance issues in social, educational, or work settings. Symptoms are divided into categories of inattention, hyperactivity, and impulsivity.

Benzodiazepines: A class of drugs that act as tranquilizers and are primarily used for treating anxiety. They also are effective in treating several other conditions, including panic attacks, seizures (convulsions), and insomnia.

Bipolar disorder: Commonly known as *bipolar affective disorder* and originally known as *manic depression*, bipolar disorder is characterized by radical shifts in mood. The elevated highs and low lows can last days or weeks at a time.

Blackout: Not to be confused with "passing out," a blackout involves a period of amnesia (memory loss) due to alcohol or drug abuse without loss of consciousness.

Borderline personality disorder: A mental disorder marked by impairments in personality and behaviors, and by the presence of pathological personality characteristics.

Cannabis: A substance typically known as *marijuana*.

Chronic: Concerning a disease, *chronic* means persisting for a long time or constantly recurring.

Codependence (codependency, codependent): This is a condition of heavy reliance on another person. It is typically characterized by an individual who is attached to a dysfunctional, one-sided relationship. The other person, the "key player," could be the codependent's spouse, partner, friend, family member, boss, or work colleague. Codependence on another keeps the disease of addiction active. In terms of processed food addiction, the codependent is called a *Processed-Food-Anonic*, similar to an *Al-Anonic*. The codependent is preoccupied with meeting the other's emotional and self-esteem needs; this is known as *other's esteem*. When the codependent does all they can to fix, help, control, empathize, or mollycoddle the addict, they become well known for their caring, saintly, angelic, and loving nature. In reality, they need this esteem from others to feel wanted, needed, and loved themselves. This is the anesthetizing effect a codependent person chases. This control of the person or the substance and the chase of the effects is analogous to a processed food addict or an alcoholic chasing the effect component of the addiction. Most importantly, the codependent, too, can and does recover from the disease of addiction.

Cognitive behavioral therapy (CBT): A form of psychotherapy that prioritizes the crucial role of thinking in how we feel and the actions we take, with a structured and directive approach. Simply stated, a CBT therapist educates their clients *how* to do, rather than telling their clients *what* to do.

Comorbidity and **comorbid**: These are common medical terms referring to the presence of one or more additional conditions or diseases co-occurring with a primary condition in the same person at the same time. Many individuals with an addiction have a coexisting mental health condition, for example, bipolar disorder.

Craving as an allergy: The phenomenon of craving as an allergy is a predisposition of restlessness, irritability, and discontentment that precedes a desire beyond the addict's physical and mental control. A complete absence of willpower in any given circumstance is a notable physiological characteristic of a craving. Giving in to this craving, the addict ingests the processed food again. What immediately follows is a return to a state of calmness—for a time, until they again experience the same restlessness, irritability, and discontentment. Once again, the craving kicks in and overrides everything that is important to them, and they ingest again. This is repeated over and over until the processed food addict can experience a psychic change.

Depressive disorder: A mood disorder characterized by persistent feelings of sadness, worthlessness, and loss of interest. It can interfere with an individual's daily functioning.

Disease: A disease is an abnormal condition that affects the organ, part, structure, or system of the body, preventing the body or the mind from working normally. Broadly speaking, the term *disease* refers to any condition that causes pain, distress, dysfunction, or death in the individual who is afflicted.

DSM: An abbreviation for the *Diagnostic and Statistical Manual of Mental Disorders*, published by the American Psychiatric Association. It provides clinicians with official definitions of, and criteria for diagnosing, mental disorders and dysfunctions. The 2013 edition of the DSM is the **DSM-5**.

Freshman 15: Typically used in the United States to refer to the weight gained during a student's first year at college—15 lb. In Australia and New Zealand, it is sometimes referred to as *first year fatties*, *fresher spread*, or *fresher five*, the latter referring to a 5-kg. gain.

Guarded prognosis: Also known as a *guarded condition*, this is a prognosis given by a practitioner when the outcome of a patient's illness is in doubt.

Holistic: From an addiction perspective, a holistic approach takes into consideration biological, psychological, social, and spiritual factors in the whole person, rather than just concentrating on the physical symptoms of a disease.

Huffing: A term used for inhalant abuse. Individuals intentionally inhale chemical vapors, such as paint thinners, paint removers, gas, glue, or spray paint, to feel a "high," or a euphoric effect. A huffing addiction is similar to an alcohol or drug addiction.

Inhalants: The various substances individuals take *only* by inhaling.

Insider: In an addiction context, and specifically in my case as an addictionologist, this term refers to my being an insider. I not only understand and know the disease of processed food addiction academically and professionally, but I also know and understand it from a personal point of view, having experienced the disease in all its varied manifestations myself.

Manifestation: As a medical definition, manifestations (also known as *symptoms*) are the signs indicating an underlying disease, for example, abdominal pains, fever, headache, cravings, constipation, diarrhea, and uncharacteristic behaviors.

Morbidity: The condition and occurrence of illness or disease in an individual. One morbidity may lead to another morbidity, which is then referred to as a **comorbidity**.

Morphine-like effects: Morphine's most striking characteristic is its analgesic effect, which is used in treating complex pain. Hence the phrase *morphine-like effects* refers to a substance that takes away chronic pain, which in addiction can be mental and/or physical pain.

Mortality: In medical terms, *mortality* is the condition of being dead. Typically, mortality is heard in terms of the number of deaths in a population over time, either in general or due to a specific cause.

Obesogenic: Typically, *obesogenic* refers to anything that promotes or contributes to obesity. Obesogenic factors include exorbitant food intake, a sedentary lifestyle, and diets rich in processed foods.

Opioids: Also known as *narcotics*, opioids are a family of substances that can be in prescription medications (painkillers) or "street drugs," such as heroin. Primarily, opioids act on the opioid receptors in the body's cells to produce morphine-like effects. They are used for pain relief, including anesthesia.

Obsessive-compulsive disorder (OCD): The presence of recurrent and persistent thoughts, urges, or impulses that are experienced as intrusive and unwanted, and which in most individuals cause marked anxiety or distress.

Post-traumatic stress disorder (PTSD): A mental disorder stemming from an individual's experience with one or more traumatic events. Typically, individuals experience a range of mental, emotional, physical, and behavioral responses after trauma, but the majority of these individuals recover naturally from the initial symptoms. However, those demonstrating PTSD symptoms—nightmares, flashbacks, panic attacks, heightened anxiety, and so on—may find the symptoms recur and continue for more than a month after the traumatic experience.

Predisposition: Typically used in the context of a *genetic predisposition*, also called a *genetic susceptibility*. It refers to an increased likelihood of developing a particular disease based on an individual's genetic makeup. It is a genetic force that might manifest certain health problems.

Prognosis: The forecast of the probable outcome or course of a disease; the patient's chance of recovery.

Psychic change: A psychic change occurs in an individual who was once guided by irrational ideas, emotions, and attitudes. They experience a profound change in body, mind, and spirit, allowing them to adopt an entirely new set of conceptions and motives that are now the guiding force behind their new substance-free lifestyle. Said another way, the person who was once hopeless begins to understand and accept they have a disease that has to be treated on a daily basis. The change causes them to willingly take responsibility for their disease.

Recovery: In recovery, individuals process a change through which they improve their health and wellness, live a self-directed life, and strive to reach their full potential. This definition is based on a new working definition of *recovery* released by the Substance Abuse and Mental Health Services Administration.

Relapse: As a chronic disease, addiction is subject to periods of relapse, a process in which an individual who has established abstinence from the substance experiences recurrence of signs and symptoms of active addiction. During the recovery process, an individual may stop treating their disease and decide not to follow the instructions given, leading to their exposure to certain triggers and other risk factors that increase the risk of returning to ingesting, using, or drinking once again. The continual treatment of the disease on a daily basis is the panacea for avoiding a relapse. I am in line with the medical model that views addiction like any other disease: a patient returns to a state of sickness after a period of remission.

Remission: Recovery from the disease of processed food addiction means the addict has been released from the physical allergy and mental obsession that underpins their addiction. Their disease is no longer active, as they treat it on a daily basis; hence, the disease of PFA is in remission. The person undergoes a change in thought, feeling, and behavior. Their old attitudes, ideas, and emotions, which were guided and underpinned by active addiction, are cast to one side, because they accept they have a disease that has to be treated on a daily basis. This enables a new set of conceptions and motives to become operative, creating a new norm; each day the person learns how to live a lifestyle that continually partakes in active recovery.

Serenity: The state of being serene, calm, tranquil, and having peace of mind.

Sobriety: Sobriety is permanent abstinence from an addictive substance with a sustained commitment to treat the disease of addiction on a daily basis, moving toward a fuller life experience. In sobriety, an individual seeks balance in the biological, psychological, social, and spiritual aspects of their health and well-being.

Substance abuse. Refers to an individual's pattern of continued substance use that often interferes with their relations with family, friends, and society at large.

See the DSM-5 for further clarification regarding addiction medicine terms and criteria for diagnosing mental disorders and dysfunctions.

Bibliography

Al-Anon Family Group Headquarters, Inc. Staff. (1986). *Al-Anon's Twelve Steps and Twelve Traditions*. New York: Al-Anon.

Alcoholics Anonymous World Services, Inc. (1980). *Dr. Bob and the Good Oldtimers*. USA: Alcoholics Anonymous World Services, Inc.

Alcoholics Anonymous. (1939). *The Big Book*. New York: World Services, Inc.

—. (1988). *Twelve Steps and Twelve Traditions* (38th ed.). New York: World Services, Inc.

Allen, J. (undated). *As a Man Thinketh*. New York: The Peter Pauper Press, Inc.

American Psychiatric Association (2013). *Diagnostic and Statistical Manual of Mental Disorders* (5th ed.). Washington, DC: American Psychiatric Publishing.

American Society of Addiction Medicine (Adoption date: April 12, 2011). *Public Policy Statement: Definition of Addiction*. www.ASAM.org.

American Temperance Society. (1835). Permanent temperance documents of the American Temperance Society. Boston: S. Bliss. Retrieved from: catalog.hathitrust.org/Record/000500689

Beattie, M. (1988). *Co-Dependent No More: How to Stop Controlling Others and Start Caring for Yourself*. New York: Harper & Row.

Beck J. S., & Beck, A. T. (2011). *Cognitive Behavior Therapy: Basics and Beyond* (2nd ed.). New York: Guilford Press.

Bill W. (1944). *The Language of the Heart: Bill W.'s Grapevine Writings.* New York: AA Grapevine.

Bradshaw, J. (1988). *Bradshaw On: The Family.* Deerfield Beach, FL: Health Communications, Inc.

Brownell, K. D., & Warner, K. E. (2009). "The perils of ignoring history: Big tobacco played dirty and millions died. How similar is big food?" *The Milbank Quarterly,* 87, 259-294. doi. org/10.1111/j.1468-0009.2009.00555.x

Bruinsma K., & Taren, D. L. (1999). "Chocolate: food or drug?" *Journal American Diet Association.* 99,1249-1256. doi. org/10.1016/S0002-8223(99)00307-7

Corsica, J. A., & Pelchat, M. L. (2010). "Food addiction: true or false?" *Current Opinion in Gastroenterology,* 26, 165-169.

da Costa Louzada, M. L. et al. (2015). "Consumption of ultra-processed foods and obesity in Brazilian adolescents and adults." *Preventive Medicine,*81, 9-15. doi.org/10.1016/j.ypmed.2015.07.018

Food Addicts Anonymous. (1987) Food Addict Anonymous Official Website. Food Addicts Anonymous. Retrieved from: https://www.foodaddictsanonymous.org/

Ford, B. & Chase. C. (1987). *Betty: A Glad Awakening.* Garden City, NY: Doubleday.

Ganter, M. (2005). *Spirituality and the Healthy Mind: Science, Therapy, and the Need for Personal Meaning.* New York: Oxford University Press Inc.

Gearhardt, A. N., Corbin, W. R., & Brownell, K. D. (2016). Development of the Yale Food Addiction Scale version 2. *Psychology of Addictive Behaviors,* 30, 113-121. doi.org/10.1037/adb0000136

Goldberg, L. (2003). "Between the Sheets: The History of Overeaters Anonymous and Its Food Plans." Retrieved from: greysheeters.blogspot.com/p/history-of-oa-grey-sheetpart-4.html

Hazelden Foundation, Inc. (1957). *The Little Red Book*. Center City, MN: Hazelden.

Hazelden Foundation, Inc. (1980). *Twenty-Four Hours a Day*. Center City, MN: Hazelden.

Hebebrand, J., Albayrak, Ö., Ada R., Antel., J, Dieguez, C., de Jong J., et al. (2014). "'Eating addiction,' rather than 'food addiction,' better captures addictive-like eating behavior." *Neuroscience Biobehavior Reviews, 47,* 295-306. doi.org/10.1016/j.neubiorev.2014.08.016

Ifland, J., Preuss, H. G., Marcus, M. T., Rourke, K. M., Taylor, W. C., Burau, K., & Manso, G. (2009). "Refined food addiction: A classic substance use disorder." *Medical Hypotheses, 72,* 518-526.

James, W. (2004). *The Varieties of Religious Experience*. USA: Barnes and Noble, Inc.

Jellinek, E. M. (1960). *The Disease Concept of Alcoholism*. New Brunswick, N.J.: United Printing Services, Inc.

Johnson, V. (1980). *I'll Quit Tomorrow*. New York: Harper & Row.

Jung, C. G., In Jaffé, A., Winston, R., & Winston, C. (1989). *Memories, Dreams, Reflections*. New York: Vintage Books.

Leshner, A. (1987). "Addiction is a brain disease, and it matters." *Science, 278,* 807-808.

Moodie, R., Stuckler, D., Monteiro, C., Sheron, N., Neal, B., Thamarangsi, T. (2013). "Profits and pandemics: prevention of harmful effects of tobacco, alcohol, and ultra-processed food and drink industries." *Lancet,* 670-679. doi.org/10.1016/S0140-6736(12)62089-3

Moubarac, J. C., Parra, D. C., Cannon, G., & Monteiro, C. A. (2014). "Food classification systems based on food processing: significance and implications for policies and actions: a systematic literature review and assessment." *Current Obesity Report, 3,* 256–272. doi.org/:10.1007/s13679-014-0092-0

Pivarunas, B., & Conner, B. T. (2015). "Impulsivity and emotion dysregulation as predictors of food addiction." *Eating Behaviors, 19,* 9-14. doi.org/10.1016/j.eatbeh.2015.06.007

Puhl, R. M., & Heuer, C. A. (2010). "Obesity stigma: Important considerations for public health." *American Journal Public Health.* 100, 1019–1028. doi.org/10.2105/AJPH.2009.159491

Raymond, K-L, Kannis-Dymand, L., Lovell, G. P. (2016). "A graduated food addiction classification approach significantly differentiates obesity among people with type 2 diabetes." *Journal Health Psychology*, 1-9.

Rogers, B. (2005). *Twenty-Five Words: How the Serenity Prayer Can Save Your Life.* San Francisco: Redwheelweiser.

Schulte, E. M., Avena, N. M., & Gearhardt, A. N. (2015). "Which foods may be addictive? The roles of processing, fat content, and glycemic load." *PLOS/ONE.* doi.org/10.1371/journal.pone.0117959

Stuckler, D., McKee, M., Ebrahim, S. & Basu, S. (2012). "Manufacturing epidemics: The role of global producers in increased consumption of unhealthy commodities including processed foods, alcohol, and tobacco." *PLOS.* doi.org/10.1371/journal.pmed.1001235

Twerski, A. J. (1982). *It Happens to Doctors, Too.* Center City, MN: Hazelden.

Vaillant, G. E. (1995). *The Natural History of Alcoholism Revisited.* Cambridge, MA: Harvard University Press.

Webster, E. A. (1970). *Our Devilish Alcoholic Personalities.* Center City, MN: Hazelden.

Wilson, B. (1957). *Alcoholics Anonymous Comes of Age.* Oxford: Harper.

Witkiewitz, K., Marlatt, G. A. & Walker, D. (2005). "Mindfulness-based relapse prevention for alcohol and substance use disorders." *Journal of Cognitive Psychotherapy: An International Quarterly*, 19, 211-228.

World Health Organization (2018) "Obesity and Overweight." Geneva: WHO. Accessed January 2018. www.who.int/news-room/fact-sheets/detail/obesity-and-overweight

About the Author

Well, this is me *and* this is my debut book. I go to bed each night as a processed food addict, and I wake up every morning as a recovered processed food addict. I attend work daily, where I am on the coalface working clinically with those at various stages of recovery from processed food addiction (and addictions to other substances). In my work I help my patients to realize they too can get well and live fulfilling lives—be happy, joyous, and free. Once I accepted I had the disease of processed food addiction, approximately twenty-five years ago now, I set about learning everything I could about it. I have studied social and behavioral science, counseling, and psychology at undergraduate and postgraduate levels. I continue to research this disease academically, while I aspire to attract subsidies, research aid, and further resources in the future so I can continue with the empirical validations that are so much needed in this new and evolving domain of addiction. I am now at the forefront of those explaining to the world that processed foods are addictive and dangerous—not only to our health but to our livelihood. I will soon be working on my next book for those who are living in denial. Stay tuned.

I will now share with you my academic, professional work bio. In short, *this is me*, all of me; may our paths cross one day.

- PhD in the domain of processed food addiction (PFA)

- BA in social science (psychology), with honors (1st class), from the University of the Sunshine Coast, Australia
- BA in behavioral science (psychology) from the Queensland University of Technology
- Diploma in counseling, plus certificates three and four in counseling, from the Counseling College of Australia

My continued research focuses on the concept of processed food addiction being a neurobiochemical condition of the brain—a bio-psycho-social-spiritual malady underpinned by a physical allergy and mental obsession. Prevention and treatment of processed food addiction is analogous to treating other addictive diseases such as alcoholism and drug addiction. Through treatment based on abstinence from the addictive substance (processed foods) processed food addicts can live happy and healthy lives.

Over the last twenty years, I have gained significant clinical experience in effectively treating alcoholism, drug addictions (stimulants, depressants, nicotine, narcotics), and processed food addiction, with a focus on permanent recovery and a contented, useful life. I am the clinical director of Karren-Lee Addictionology, an expanding addictions practice. Importantly, I have specialized in the treatment of processed food addiction for the last fifteen-plus years, observing more often than not that it is comorbid with other substances, including alcohol, marijuana, and cocaine.

Being a pioneer in specifically treating processed food addiction, I conduct workshops for professionals and processed food addicts both in Australia and internationally. In 2018 I presented my latest research in the processed food addiction arena at the International Society of Addiction Medicine (ISAM) in South Korea. In the past I have also attended and presented research on processed food addiction at other ISAM conferences, including ISAM 2017 Abu Dhabi and the Joint ISAM Conference: ISAM and CSAM-SMCA XXVII (the Canadian Society of Addiction Medicine). I received a scholarship to fund my attendance and presentations at this annual-meeting-plus-scientific-conference in Montreal in 2016. I continue to present yearly at Processed Food Addiction Workshops in Baltimore and to work with international patients several times a year, traveling to their countries of residence.

Additionally, I am the founder of the Annual Karren-Lee Addictionology Processed Food Addictions Retreat, held every February in Brisbane since 2012. This is supported by several national and international workshops and webinars for those seeking recovery and for those who have recovered from processed food addiction and addictions to other substances throughout the years. I am professionally affiliated with the societies of addiction medicine in Canada and the US, and with the international societies: CSAM-SMCA, ASAM, and ISAM.

Lastly, I have collaborated with, met, and received guidance from many professionals and organizations, including Diabetes Australia, Diabetes UK, and Diabetes Ireland. I continue to do post-doctorate research with Associate Professor Geoff Lovell, PhD, and a team of researchers at home here in Australia, and I look forward to international collaboration in the research arena in the future.

In conclusion, I share with you recently published innovative research in the processed food realm, with further international research projects in the stages of collation of data and analysis, as well as written manuscripts in review that are awaiting publication.

Contact

Karren-Lee Raymond, PhD, ISAM CSAM-SMCA CHI ASAM

karren-lee@addictionology.com.au

Recent Publications

Raymond, K-L., & Lovell, G. P. (2015). "Food addiction symptomology, impulsivity, mood, and body mass index in people with type two diabetes." *Appetite*, 95, 383-389. doi.org/10.1016/j.appet.2015.07.030

Raymond, K-L., & Lovell, G. P. (2016). "Food addiction associations with psychological distress among people with type 2 diabetes." *Journal of Diabetes and its Complications*, 30, 651-656. doi.org/10.1016/j.jdiacomp.2016.01.020

Raymond, K-L., Kannis-Dymand, L., & Lovell, G. P. (2016). "A graduated food addiction classification approach significantly differentiates obesity among people with type 2 diabetes." *Journal of Health Psychology*, 1-10. doi.org/10.1177/1359105316672096

Raymond, K-L., Kannis-Dymand, L., & Lovell, G. P. (2017). "A Graduated food addiction classifications approach significantly differentiates depression, anxiety and stress among people with type 2 diabetes." *Diabetes Research and Clinical Practice*. 132, 95-101. doi.org/10.1016/j.diabres.2017.07.028

www.ingramcontent.com/pod-product-compliance
Lightning Source LLC
Chambersburg PA
CBHW020856020526
44107CB00076B/1872